PSILOCYBIN MUSHROOMS

A Step-by-Step Guide on How to Grow and Safely Use Psychedelic Magic Mushrooms for Beginners

MARC PETERSON

© **Copyright 2021 - All rights reserved.**

The content contained within this book may not be reproduced, duplicated or transmitted without direct written permission from the author or the publisher.

Under no circumstances will any blame or legal responsibility be held against the publisher, or author, for any damages, reparation, or monetary loss due to the information contained within this book, either directly or indirectly.

Legal Notice:

This book is copyright protected. It is only for personal use. You cannot amend, distribute, sell, use, quote, or paraphrase any part, or the content within this book, without the consent of the author or publisher.

Disclaimer Notice:

Please note the information contained within this document is for educational and entertainment purposes only. All effort has been executed to present accurate, up to date, reliable, complete information. No warranties of any kind are declared or implied. Readers acknowledge that the author is not engaged in the rendering of legal, financial, medical or professional advice. The content within this book has been derived from various sources. Please consult a licensed professional before attempting any techniques outlined in this book.

By reading this document, the reader agrees that under no circumstances is the author responsible for any losses, direct or indirect, that are incurred as a result of the use of the information contained within this document, including, but not limited to, errors, omissions, or inaccuracies.

PSILOCYBIN MUSHROOMS

Table of Contents

Introduction vii

Chapter 1: Psilocybin Mushrooms - What and Why 1

  Origins 2

    Evolution Of Fungi 2

    The Network 5

    Growth 7

    The History Of Psilocybin 8

    Recent History 19

  The Benefits 21

    Depression Treatment 23

    Ptsd 25

    Addiction Treatment 26

    Psychological Distress 27

    Spiritual Progression 27

    Creativity And Art 30

  Why This Matters 31

Chapter 2: The Right Mushroom for You 32

  What To Expect 33

    Spore Availability 34

    Natural Availability 34

    Cultivability 35

    Potency 36

    Uses 37

    Individual Experience 39

PSILOCYBIN MUSHROOMS

    Psychoactive Mushroom Species 40

        Amanita Muscaria 41

        Psilocybe Allenii 44

        Psilocybe Azurescens 47

        Psilocybe Caerulescens 49

        Psilocybe Caerulipes 50

        Psilocybe Cubensis 51

        Psilocybe Cyanescens 53

        Psilocybe Mexicana 54

        Psilocybe Semilanceata 57

        Psilocybe Stuntzii 59

        Psilocybe Tampanensis 60

    Have You Decided? 61

Chapter 3: Cultivating Psilocybin Mushrooms 64

    Where To Grow 64

        Outside 65

        Indoors 67

    Getting Started 68

        Terminology 69

    Cultivation Methods And Substrates 72

        Pick A Substrate 73

        Decide On A Fruiting Chamber Setup 80

    A Step-By-Step Guide 87

        Monotub And Grain Spawn Method 88

        Shotgun Fruiting Chamber(Sgfc) And Cake Method .. 104

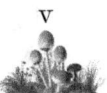

- Outside Cultivation With Grain Spawn ... 120
- Building A Greenhouse ... 124
- It Is Not That Difficult ... 130

Chapter 4: Harvesting and Storage ... 132

- The Harvesting Process ... 132
  - Precautions ... 133
  - Harvesting Your Mushrooms ... 135
  - Continue Growing ... 138
- Making Your Own Spore Kits ... 139
  - Spore Prints ... 140
  - Spore Syringes ... 142
- Storing Your Mushrooms ... 143
  - Fresh Storage ... 146
  - Drying ... 147
  - Other Methods Of Storage ... 149
- That's It! ... 150

Chapter 5: Using Psilocybin Mushrooms Safely ... 152

- Magic Mushroom Dosage Guide ... 153
- Different Consumption Methods ... 156

Chapter 6: General Tips ... 159

- Pest, Contamination, And Disease Control ... 159
  - Pests ... 159
  - Contamination And Disease ... 162
- Some Tips ... 164

Conclusion ... 166

INTRODUCTION

Psilocybin mushrooms—how does one go about cultivating them by oneself? More importantly, what is the safest way to enjoy the fruits of your labor? These two questions have been frequently asked over the last few years. This is most likely due to the exponential rise in the popularity of psychedelics; however, with such a rise in popularity, the demand for psychedelic substances has risen as well.

This has made psychedelic mushrooms one of the go-to first tries for many people, be it just for the experience itself or the self-sufficiency. But the experience of becoming completely self-sufficient in producing a natural form of psychedelics is the ultimate goal after all.

Psilocybin mushrooms can be found in nature, occurring in many shapes, forms, and species, so you do not necessarily have to grow your own. The problem is not everyone is experienced enough to identify the correct ones, so you might end up poisoning yourself. This leaves you with two other options—either find someone trustworthy who will sell you some or cultivate your own.

While the former is still an option, the latter is something more than just enjoying a psychedelic experience.

Cultivating and consuming your own psilocybin

mushrooms is very rewarding in its own way.

Most of you reading this will have had a psychedelic experience before. How else would you even begin to understand the importance or value in cultivating for yourself? However, there are some people who can spot the benefits before even having an experience themselves. For those of you who have not had such an experience before, no problem! You can start yourself off the right way. I could only imagine the thrill in having your first experience be one from your own labor.

I would usually suggest to most people to try psilocybin mushrooms at least once before cultivating their own. But over the years, this opinion has changed. While this is not a must, however, since growing my own I have come to realize the importance of producing your own stock.

Not everyone is ready to jump into such a commitment yet though, so trying some first with a friend or two will also help you determine if it actually is for you.

Not everyone enjoys the experience these fungi can provide them with. While this may simply be due to personal preference, it can happen due to consuming bad shrooms. A bad first experience with mushrooms can occur with anyone, even when you had good previous experiences. What's worse is a bad first experience might put you off from any future psychedelic trips, which might have changed your life in a positive manner.

In this book, we will be taking a look at how you can

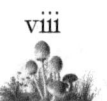

cultivate, harvest, and store your own magic mushrooms efficiently. Not only that, but we will also go over how to safely use your mushrooms. This will lower the chance of ever having a bad experience, especially the former. Using psilocybin safely will lead to a great many benefits as well, which we will of course discuss later on. Realizing the benefits of consuming them can sometimes come too late, so in this book, we will go over health, mental, emotional, and spiritual benefits.

Firstly, you will have to understand mushrooms, or fungi, a little better in order to cultivate them. We will discuss in depth the rich history of psilocybin mushrooms, through which you can gain a better understanding of all their applicable uses. Learning the origin of fungi will make it so much easier to cultivate magic mushrooms, as you will understand the fundamentals of their existence.

It's like building a house—you cannot skip the foundations.

While we go through some of the popular species, you can decide on the type of shroom you will want to cultivate. It will be important when looking into what type of experience you want to have, as well as the availability of spores in your area.

Growing and cultivating your own psilocybin mushrooms is not that difficult, and it can be done in a great many ways. We will be taking a look at all the possible ways, so you can decide on what method works for you!

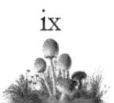

Whether you have decided to cultivate your own psilocybin mushrooms or not, yet, this book is here to help you out!

CHAPTER 1

PSILOCYBIN MUSHROOMS - WHAT AND WHY

With so many psychedelic substances currently out in the world, people are confused. Which one is the best one? What is the difference between them? Are the experiences different? You can rest easy, however, as I will explain to you why psychedelic mushrooms are the best option for you.

Magic mushrooms are one of the best options for a first psychedelic experience overall. The experience it provides can range from simple open-mindedness or acute focus, to a full-on trip. The naturally occurring mushroom, compared to a fabricated psychedelic like LSD, is a more trustworthy substance for many.

The experience is usually shorter than LSD as well. The typical psychedelic experience from magic mushrooms can

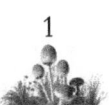

last between two to six hours, depending on the dosage. LSD, however, can last between eight to 14 hours. This makes shrooms the best option for beginners. Should a bad trip be experienced, or simply a very vibrant or overwhelming trip, it won't last too long.

Now that you understand why psilocybin mushrooms are the best option, you will have to understand mushrooms in order to cultivate them. Let us explore the origin and history of magic mushrooms.

Origins

Many people do not believe it is important to understand the way fungi, or mushrooms, work. While it is true that you do not need a complex understanding of how the cellular structure of fungi works, it is still necessary to have a basic understanding. When you grow your own, you will come to realize that simply following a few steps in order to sprout some magic mushrooms will work.

However, when you want to focus on actually growing quality mushrooms, experiment a bit with different methods, and add your own ingenious techniques, you will need to understand how they are formed.

So, let's start at the very beginning.

Evolution of Fungi

The evolution of the magic mushroom starts out with basic fungi. It all began 1.5 billion years ago when the fungus itself diverged from all other life. The earliest fossils of life presenting basic fungi features were discovered to be around 1 billion years old.

At around 400–500 million years ago, fungi began growing their own network around the world. This network is known as mycelium. Many people know mycelium as just the early vegetative state of fungus, before the fruiting bodies, or mushrooms, grow from it. You can imagine mycelium as roots to a tree. While they might not function exactly the same, fungi use mycelium to draw in nutrients.

Fungi were the first form of flora on planet Earth, way before other vegetation started to grow. Shortly after the appearance of fungus came nonvascular plants, however. By around 300 million years ago, all modern forms of fungus were present. Now think about that for a second—while many new species of fungus have been discovered, the base form has not changed for 300 million years. Fungi do not have the need to evolve any further. In fact, there are forms of fungus that can survive out in the vacuum of space and forms that survive simply by feeding on radiation.

PSILOCYBIN MUSHROOMS

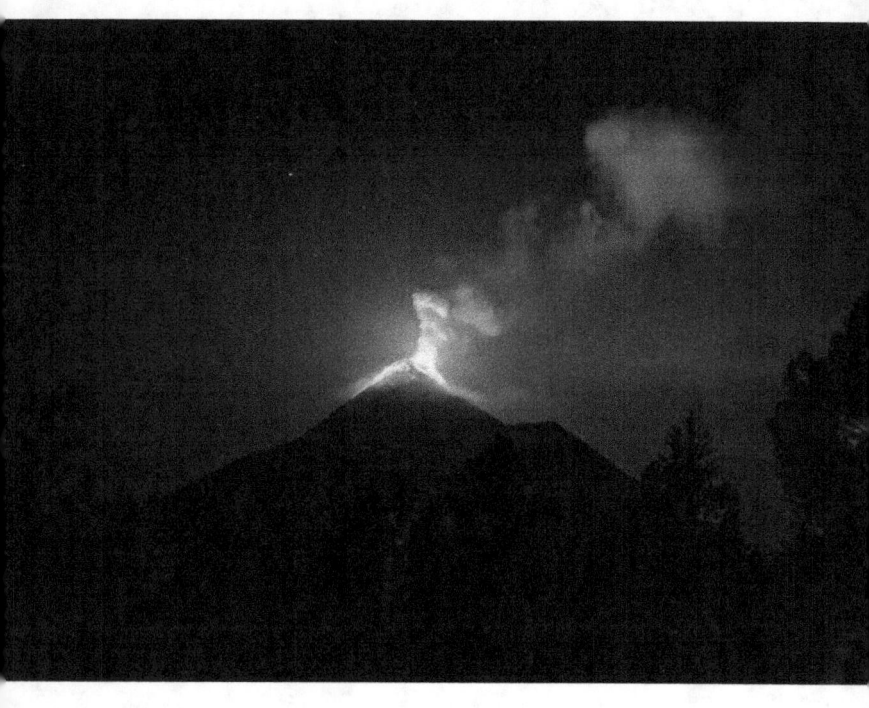

Fungi were so perfect of an organism that it became the dominant species around the world for a long time. After what is known as the Permian - Triassic extinction event 251 million years ago, a dramatic spike in what was thought to be fungal spores was seen. However, this extinction event is known as the Earth's most severe one, which wiped out about 80% of marine life and 70% of land animals. That means the dominant species was fungi. The fossil records for this period have a 100% representation of fungi species.

These discoveries have led to many legitimate hypotheses as well as many other theories, which we will get into later.

It is believed that the reason the fungus has survived so long is due to mycelium. This network of fungi led to the perfect way of exchanging information.

The Network

Mycelia can be seen as a massive network in the soil making up the floor of forests. While it doesn't appear only in forests, it is the best example to use, in order to explain just how amazing mycelium is.

You will be experiencing mycelium firsthand, working with it closely. It is a good idea to understand more about it, so let's go over a few things.

In a forest-like environment, trees and plants communicate, using mycelium as a network. It is essentially their internet. When I heard about this network

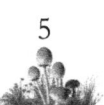

for the first time, I did not think much of it—I mean what can mushrooms and plants even communicate about?

In a forest, many trees and plants will grow to different sizes. This can happen due to a lack of nutrients and so the mycelium network gets accessed. It is through this network the plants and trees will spread information to each other. Plants not getting the nutrients they need will request more of it from the other trees through the network. The nutrients will then be transferred using that network in order to help some plants get the nutrient they need to survive.

Let that sink in for a minute… is it just me, or is that insanely astounding?

You see, mycelia get nutrients from plants themselves, but they do not suck them completely dry. In fact, they help plants absorb other nutrients as well as water. This relationship led mycelia to become one of the largest organisms on the planet.

Massive networks spanning hundreds of miles underground, all connected. This has led plants to communicate with each other over vast areas. It has been observed through a few studies that when certain pests or diseases start to appear in one part of a forest, the immune response of plants connected to the network will improve, whereas the plants not connected to such a network have a difficult time, as they were not prepared.

From these networks, mushrooms started spawning all over the world. The rapid pace at which different species of mushrooms pop up almost overnight has led to the belief that there are millions of different species. This rapid expansion of mushroom growth led to the birth of psilocybin mushrooms.

Growth

The actual mushrooms do not really take that long to grow. You will see later on when going over how to cultivate your own mushrooms that it doesn't take more than a month. Compared to other plants, that is very quick.

At first, growth out of mycelium starts with what is known as the fruiting body. It can take days to form this basic primordial body. They start out as small, round pins forming all over the network. This stage is known as the pin stage, as they really are tiny. Through the intake of nutrients and large amounts of water relative to their size, they move onto the button stage, expanding just slightly.

Once these stages of formation are complete, the amount of fluid and nutrient absorption rapidly increases. This serves to inflate the cells that were formed in the fruiting bodies.

Now, this process can take days; however, certain species of mushroom can pop up in a few hours and release their spores. They will be gone just as quickly as they arrived. Luckily for us, psilocybin-containing mushrooms do not disappear in a few hours. But on the other hand, that means they do not grow overnight either, so you will have to be patient.

That network of mycelia, however, does not disappear. In fact, it can stay there for years, growing fruiting bodies so long as there are nutrients and fluids. This will also be helpful when getting to grow your own.

As mentioned, these mycelium networks do not go away unless they are either destroyed or the nutrients run out. There is what can be described as a colony of mushrooms in the Malheur National Forest. This colony is kept alive by a massive network of mycelia believed to be more than 2,500 years old, spanning over a 2,200-acre area.

The History of Psilocybin

Many historians believe psilocybin mushrooms to have been used as far back as 10,000 BCE. That could mean a lot for human evolution. Before we get into that, however, let's first take a look at what history has shown us about cultivation and use.

Evidence shows that psychoactive mushrooms have been used for a long time, even before the birth of civilization as we know it, around 6,000 years ago. As mentioned, the earliest evidence that we have of mushrooms being consumed dates back to around 10,000 BCE. A mural found in northern Australia depicts images of mushrooms on the cave walls. It might not be concrete proof of the consumption of psilocybin mushrooms, but it is logical, however, to assume that they have been used from the beginning of existence of *Homo sapien*.

There are two main reasons for this premise:

1. Psilocybin mushrooms, or any mushroom for that matter, are found all over most continents. So, we can assume that hominids most likely consumed these on their journeys through the landscapes. Some might even have gained certain evolutionary advantages due to their experiences.

2. Many species still consume plants containing psychoactive substances. Dolphins consume the psychotropic toxins found on pufferfish. We all know just how intelligent and social dolphins are, so they most likely enjoy the experiences it provides. Reindeer in North America and Serbia consume the popularly depicted red-domed and white-dotted mushroom known as *Amanita muscaria*.

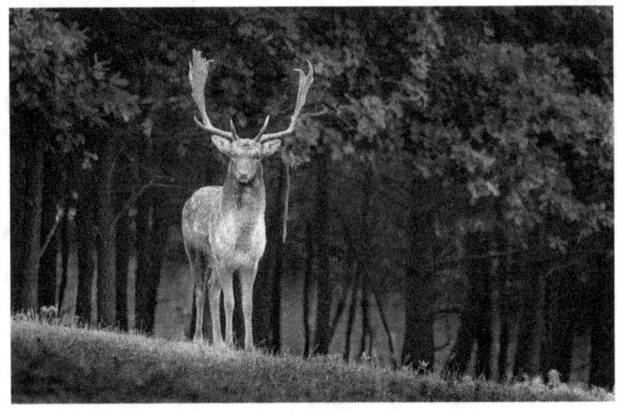

It has been observed that the deer will go to great lengths just to eat these mushrooms. They will exhibit drunken behavior, run around aimlessly, make strange noises, and twitch. So, they as well most likely do it just for enjoyment.

Jaguars consume the yage' vine, known to be a major component in the psychoactive drink ayahuasca. While it is unclear exactly why they ingest it, they have been observed to act quite strangely for a while. They will then prioritize hunting, so some people believe they consume it to sharpen their hunting reflexes.

When looking at the consumption of these substances in nature, it is not too reckless to believe that early *Homo sapiens* have also consumed these substances. In the last few years, this has led to quite a few theories regarding the evolution of the hominid species.

Terrence Mckenna is a well-known ethnobotanist, especially for his psychedelic exploits and associated stories. But many know him for his "stoned ape" theory. Considering how old these psilocybin mushrooms are, the theory could hold some promise.

PSILOCYBIN MUSHROOMS

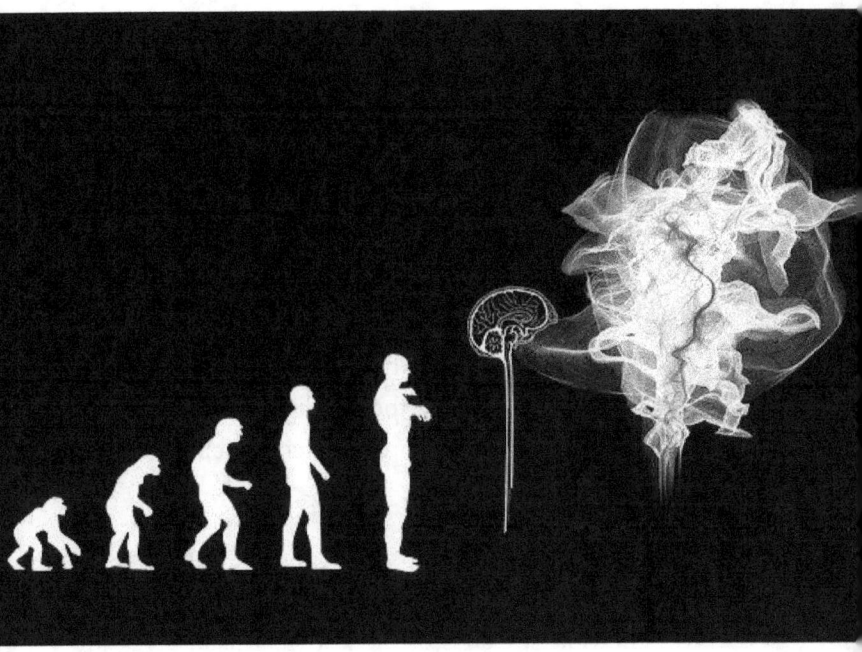

The theory postulates that while consuming these mushrooms, hominids could have been unknowingly expanding their minds. This coincides with the growth of the human brain through the years. The brain of *Homo erectus* doubled in size over a few million years, and the brain of *Homo sapien* became three times larger in the span of just a few hundred thousand years.

Terrence wrote a book named *Food of the Gods*, in which he expressed this theory. He proposed that our ancestors most likely used these mushrooms for the psychedelic visuals, as well as a boost in hunting capabilities. He proposed that by eating these substances, ancient humans expanded the capacity of their minds and the brain's processing capabilities.

While we cannot yet prove this, more studies are being conducted in order to prove the validity of this theory, as the premise becomes more and more convincing.

Moving forward in time from the evolution of *Homo sapien*, we do at least see proof of psilocybin mushrooms being used. The use of these mushrooms has been seen all over the world in tribal societies, as their depictions in caves and temples show us.

Many forms of art found in Central America, Serbia, Greece, and Egypt depict the usage of these mushrooms.

The art found in Central America, as well as the nomenclature of the Maya and Aztec people, indicates that they thought of these psilocybin mushrooms as a means of communicating with the gods. Many religious legends and myths surrounding Aztec, Maya, and Toltecs are quite full of references to these mushrooms. An example of that would be the story of how the serpent god Quetzocoatl gave these mushrooms to their ancestors. This is most likely why their word for psilocybin mushrooms translates to "flesh of the gods."

PSILOCYBIN MUSHROOMS

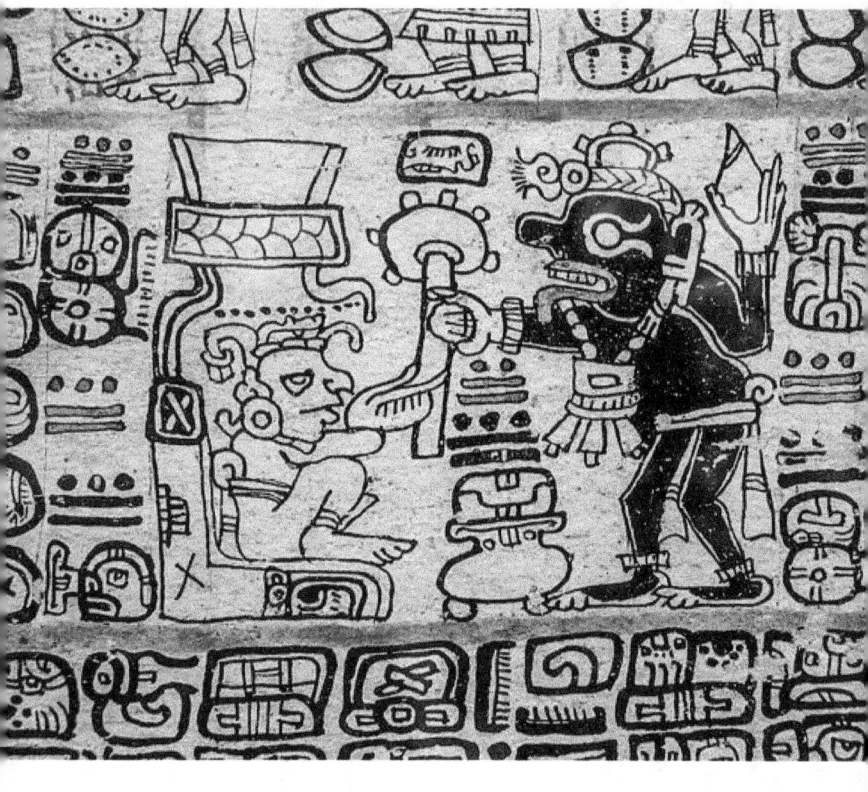

PSILOCYBIN MUSHROOMS

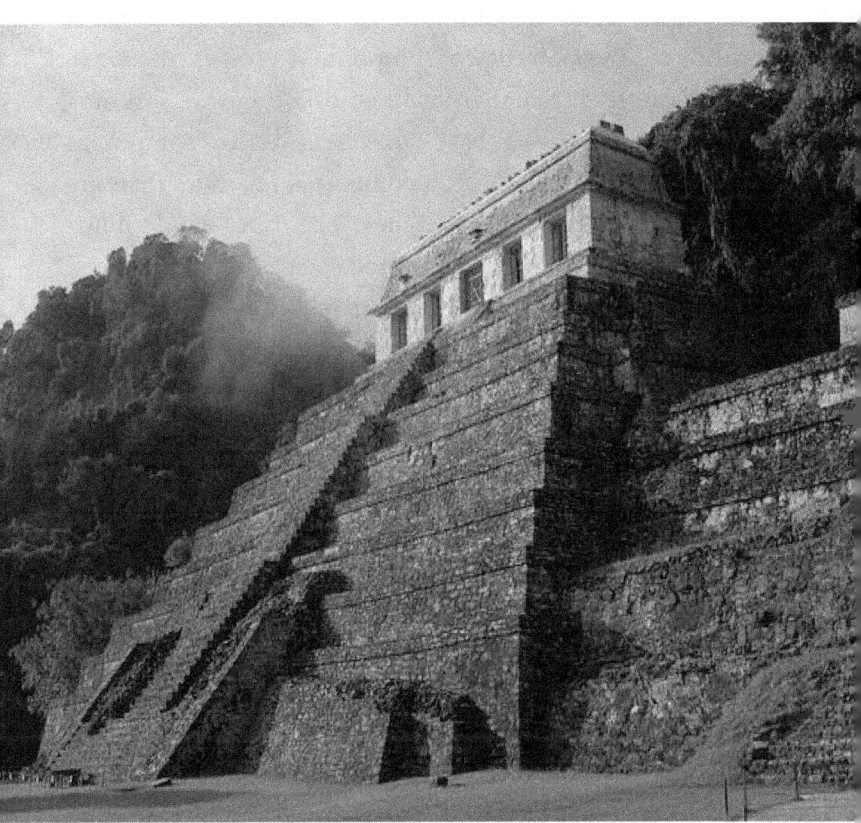

Amanita muscaria was consumed by the ancient indigenous tribes of Serbia. While it is quite dangerous to consume it as is, they found another way. The tribe would drink, and many still drink, the urine of reindeer who consumed these mushrooms. The urine is highly psychoactive and not at all toxic, as the mushroom itself can be. The experience produced through the consumption of *Amanita muscaria* is significantly different from basic psilocybin mushrooms, as *Amanita muscaria* has a different active compound, muscimol. Ultimately, it could be used for more than just a spiritual journey or experience. The tribes would utilize this mushroom to achieve altered states of consciousness, exceeding normal physical and psychological limits. They would be able to hunt and endure extreme temperatures for extended periods of time.

PSILOCYBIN MUSHROOMS

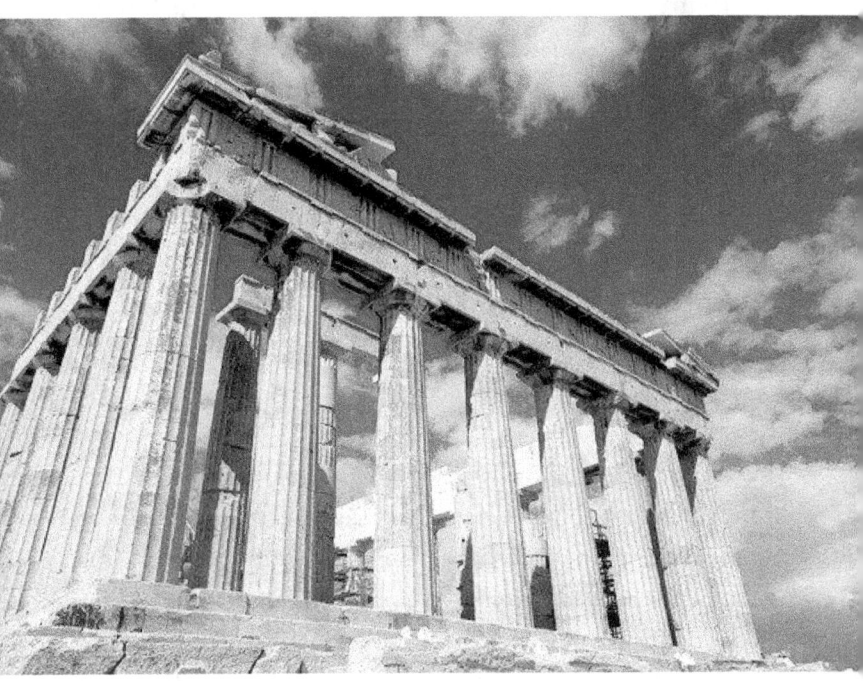

In ancient Greece, a ritual known as "The Eleusinian Mysteries" was a rebirth of sorts, through the consumption of the potion known as "kykeon." This brew was made in many forms, but psilocybin mushrooms and/or *Amanita muscaria* mushrooms would usually be the active ingredient. The ritual was meant to provide spiritual insight and healing, and as such, anyone who experienced it was sworn to secrecy. The penalty for exposing this ritual was death. Many of the intellectual Greeks and Romans like Plato, Sophocles, Cicero, and Marcus Aurelius went on the pilgrimage to Eleusis.

Eleusis was known as the spiritual capital of the world at this point.

Egyptians were also known to consume magic mushrooms, going as far as actually cultivating them on barley. They consumed a variety of these mushrooms, including *Amanita muscara* and psilocybin mushrooms. Not a lot is known about the rituals they performed with these mushrooms. It is known, however, that in *The Book of the Dead*, it is known as "celestial food."

PSILOCYBIN MUSHROOMS

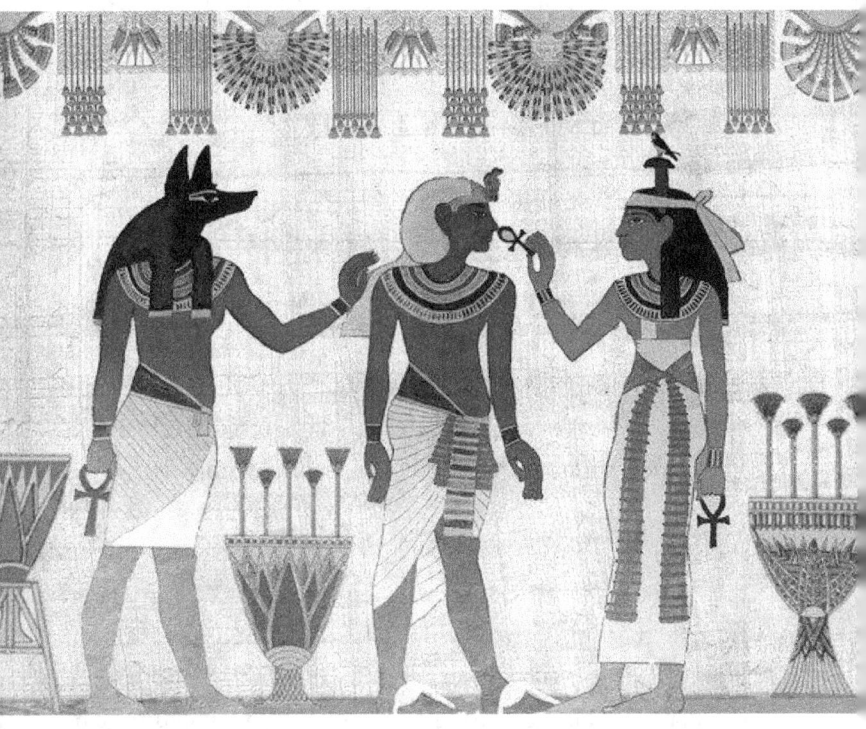

Recent History

The phrase "magic mushroom" only came to the United States around 1950. This was due to the research and findings of mycologist R. Gordon Wasson. He went to Mexico in order to conduct research on mushrooms, where he participated in a ritual ceremony led by a Mazatec shaman. After his experiences, he came back to write an article about these findings. The editor came up with the title "Seeking the Magic Mushroom."

Many got wind of this article, starting their own journeys and experimentation. A man named Albert Hofmann was the first to isolate and synthesize the active compound psilocybin.

Timothy Leary, a well-known psychologist and psychedelic advocate, was a Harvard professor at this time. He gained interest in psilocybin, leading him to travel to Mexico and participate in the ceremonies as well. Richard Alpert, a spiritual teacher, joined Leary in those expeditions. Both of these men experienced profound transformations, after which they founded the famous Harvard Psilocybin Project, a study conducted on Harvard graduate students through the use of psilocybin. The project ended in 1963 due to some ethical issues, however.

It is in this time period when Terrance McKenna and his brother Dennis traveled to the Amazon in search of DMT. What they found instead was a psilocybin-containing mushroom. After their experiences, they returned to the United States and released publications on cultivating magic mushrooms. This is what is believed to have led to a massive surge in the availability of psilocybin in the US.

This massive spike in the use of psychoactive drugs resulted in a ban on psilocybin in the 1970s.

Luckily, the spores themselves were not banned, due to the fact that they do not contain any psilocybin themselves. This made the cultivation of these mushrooms still a possibility in the future.

That future is now, with the interest in it spiking again and proper studies being approved.

These days, the acceptance of psilocybin-containing mushrooms is much wider than it was in the 20th century. As such, the number of people experimenting with it has risen dramatically. The amount being cultivated around the world is most likely incalculable, and the studies that are being approved shine a light on our future. In 2018, one of the biggest studies yet was approved by the FDA. We have come quite far.

The Benefits

When your decision to grow your own mushrooms comes into question, you can always start to focus on what the benefits might be. While many studies have been conducted, and many more will still be conducted, there are some benefits that have been realized. Perhaps it is time we discuss these benefits. Many people will claim psilocybin as a miracle drug to be used in order to cure all manner of ailments. That is simply not true. When you think about it, aren't those unrealistic expectations from one chemical compound? While it is certainly true that psilocybin can help us in many ways, we need to have patience.

At this point, we already have quite a few ways this compound helps, but more research needs to be conducted. The sudden ban on most psychoactive compounds in the 1970s brought most research to halt as well. So, while we could have been much further along, we are not. Let's have a quick look at how exactly it affects the brain. That way, we can better understand how medicinal applications might benefit us.

Early in 2020, new ground was broken when a team of scientists was able to construct a model of the human brain on psilocybin. This was achieved through a study based on brain scans from nine different participants. The participants were injected with either psilocybin or a placebo. During a set amount of time, their brains were mapped using scans and imaging to compare to the previous states. The scientists used those images and comparisons to create a "simulated brain," providing an image of all the neurons in the brain, as well as the live activity of the neurotransmitters.

During an average day, your brain fires all kinds of signals; these signals are interpreted by neurons, the cells in your brain. The neurons will carry all of this info on a selected path, while neurotransmitters will transfer those signals between neurons and their receivers—synapses.

PSILOCYBIN MUSHROOMS

Imagine a big city with cars going through intersections, following a predetermined path to GPS coordinates.

When psilocybin is introduced, however, those signals travel completely different paths, almost creating their own new network. So, those cars are not driving the predetermined path anymore; they take what way they want to.

There are a few more complicated things that happen between the neurotransmitters and the receivers, but essentially scientists have now come to realize the exact way psilocybin affects the brain. This opens further studies into using this compound in tandem with proper treatment, for more psychological, spiritual, and emotional benefits.

Depression Treatment

While studies are still being conducted, there are a few ways we can use magic mushrooms to relieve or completely treat depression. While it will depend on the person's current mental state, psilocybin can be introduced into their system so they may become more focused, energized, and confident.

When used correctly, those altered states of consciousness can enhance your insight into specific situations or previous occurrences. Coupled with therapy, depression can be overcome. There have already been many cases where people have completely dropped therapy and western medicine altogether, simply due to the fact that consuming magic mushrooms helped them in a more profound way.

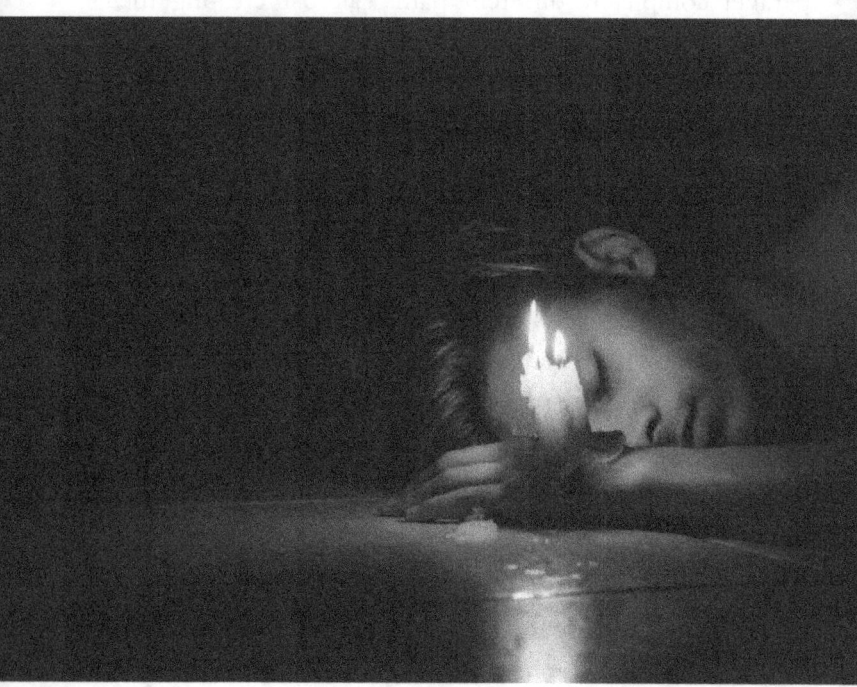

Some of these accounts come from women struggling with depression. They have had difficulty coping with the stress of work or perhaps have difficulty connecting with their kids. Through proper microdosing, these women have been able to find new motivation in life. They became more efficient at work, resulting in relieving stress and a boost in confidence. They were able to connect with their children simply due to being more energized.

Some people have claimed to have only used a recreational dose once and come out of their experience for the better. Developing a more open mindset can sometimes be just what you need in order to move on from what might be causing your depression in the first place.

PTSD

When someone consumes psilocybin, or most psychoactive substances for that matter, they will gain the ability to access their past. I do not mean time travel—I simply mean the basic access to memories or events that were once forgotten.

Your brain will seal off and block traumatic past experiences from your conscious mind. However, this can cause problems in future psychological progress.

When psilocybin is introduced, you will be able to access those memories in order to come to terms with what might have transpired. You may gain a new and more profound understanding of the event itself, enabling you to process it and psychologically put it to rest. If a properly guided session through your mind, with the use of psilocybin, is conducted professionally, the results could be very beneficial.

Most programs out there are currently 12-step recovery programs. They focus on the process of uncovering personal memories, which might be the root cause of trauma or emotional instability. This whole process can be quite time consuming and sometimes even more of a traumatic experience. When using psilocybin, however, it can be done more swiftly and to a much more balanced and further extent.

Addiction Treatment

A small study conducted at Johns Hopkins University in 2016 showed promising results in the treatment for nicotine addiction. Fifteen participants completed a 12-month follow-up after consuming psilocybin mushrooms with the objective of abstaining from smoking.

Twelve of these 15 returned again for a 16-month follow-up. At the 12-month follow-up, 10 participants were confirmed to still be abstaining from smoking. At the 16-month follow-up, nine participants were still abstaining from the use of nicotine. Thirteen of the participants said their psilocybin experiences rated in the top five of their personally meaningful and life-changing experiences.

According to the leader of the study, psilocybin has the potential to treat other substance use disorders as well, not just nicotine.

"The general idea is that the nature of these disorders is a narrowed mental and behavioral repertoire. So, [psilocybin] in well-orchestrated sessions [has] the ability to essentially shake someone out of their routine to give a glimpse of a larger picture and create a mental plasticity with which people can step outside of those problems" (Johnson et al., 2016).

Psychological Distress

The treatment for terminal cancer patients who suffer from psychological stress can be greatly improved through the use of something like magic mushrooms. When patients become depressed, psilocybin can help them deal with the existential dread they might be facing. This will of course be dependent on proper administration and counseling.

Spiritual Progression

When talking about the benefits of psilocybin-containing mushrooms, I will try to concentrate on the quantifiable, fact-based benefits. We cannot deny that factual evidence does make for a more convincing argument. However, this does not mean all benefits to the individual can be measured and studied. When going through one of these experiences, your life can change. As many of you must know, the experience can be enlightening, just as it can be terrifying. When first going on a spiritual journey, one might start out with meditation. Others might have their spiritual journey jump-started by the use of magic mushrooms. One thing, however, remains certain with all who have had the experience. They gained a profound understanding, and they had a long-term psychological benefit from that understanding.

Talking from personal experience, the first mushroom trip I had was with no intention of finding myself. I was simply having a good time with my friends, and we thought a weekend out on a farm with some shrooms could be interesting. I went in blind, with no expectations or any prior research. I came out of it, however, with a bigger picture in my head—I gained perspective.

This new-found view I had on life led me on a spiritual journey to actually start finding myself. I would argue that something so simple, but yet mind-blowing, can change the course of your future. That will cause many to look at it as terrifying, but that is not the case. When talking about spiritual progress, you have to move at your own pace. Something that might sound terrifying to you now can simply mean that you are not yet ready for the changes it might provide you with, and there is nothing wrong with that.

PSILOCYBIN MUSHROOMS

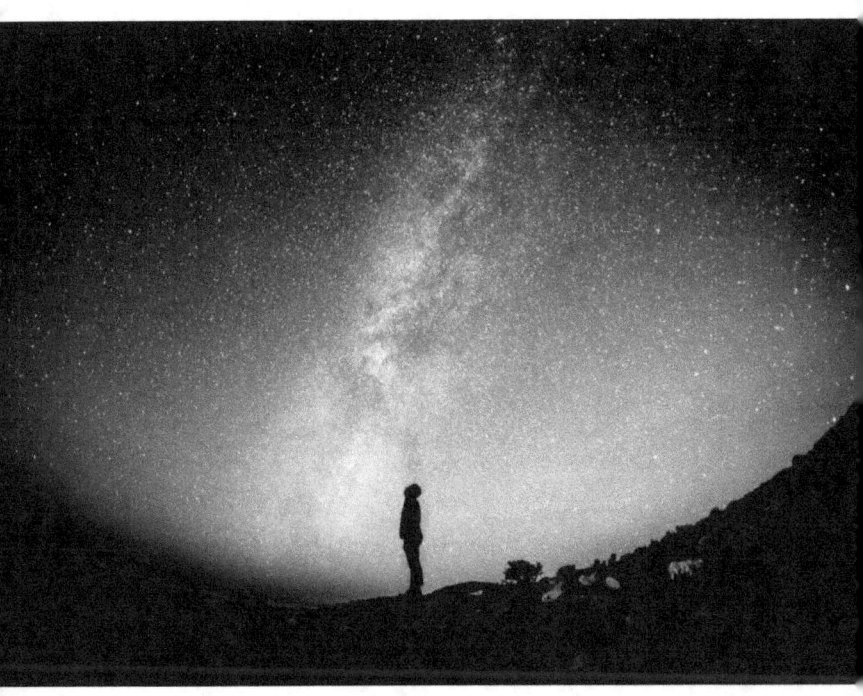

That is why I believe having more information on the subject can lead anyone to make a properly informed decision, so they may walk their own spiritual journey.

Creativity and Art

Another benefit many people seem to have forgotten in these modern times is expanding one's creative mind. In this time period, we are usually so restricted by certain beliefs, social acceptance, societal demands, and even just the stress of day-to-day life. We have forgotten how to be creative. Everything is generic these days. From the music you listen to, the shows you watch on TV, the videos on social media and YouTube, all of it follows certain rules and restrictions—many of those restrictions being the need to monetize.

When an individual feels lost or cramped in a box, a creative outlet can save their life. Magic mushrooms can help you unlock the once lost creative side of any human being. Originality can be something simple such as enjoying a hobby, building something new, writing music, painting—any form of creative expression. Cultivating magic mushrooms can even become one of those hobbies.

The benefit comes when we start exploring new parts of our minds; the creative sides will reveal themselves, and we will start creating new things. Being stuck in a generic world will become cold—humanity will need creative minds to break everyone away from mindless conformity.

It is often discussed how consciousness is connected to everything. When having a profound experience through consuming magic mushrooms, consciousness cracks open, sometimes breaking the image of the individual. It is at that point, however, that you realize the benefits of individual creativity.

Why This Matters

When dealing with magic mushrooms, it is always good to have the right mindset. Learning about how exactly they work provides you with a broader perspective before you actually start growing any.

Now you understand a bit of the history behind the cultivation and use of magic mushrooms. Learning a bit about how fungi work helps you to better understand the process of cultivating. Later, when dealing with the cultivation process step by step, you will grasp the reasons behind those steps, leading to an easier cultivation experience.

Understanding the many benefits the consumption of mushrooms can provide you with, you might be more motivated to grow them properly. Growing any type of plant or fungus is much easier when you are fully dedicated to it, rather than simply stumbling through it all.

CHAPTER 2

THE RIGHT MUSHROOM FOR YOU

When starting out, you might have an idea in your mind as to what you will be using these mushrooms for. Will you be consuming them with a few friends for recreational purposes? Will you be using them for medicinal purposes? Perhaps for psychological or spiritual use? Something that many people forget is that not every magic mushroom trip or experience will be the same.

While this will all depend on the individual in question, different strains will all provide different results. Not only may the experience itself differ, but the overall effects it will have on you mentally or physically can differ as well.

That is why it is important to do some research on what type of psilocybin mushroom you actually want to cultivate. What you might also not realize is that different species will grow a bit differently than others. This can be seen in the timeframe as well as the physical difference between them.

You will also need to know what strain is available to you in your area. It does not matter a lot, as you can grow almost any strain so long as you keep the conditions optimal. What does matter is how you will get the spores for them. Importing spores from far away can get quite costly. So, it is best to instead look for something available locally to start out with.

In this chapter, we will be going over the differences between some of the most popular species and strains of psilocybin mushrooms. We will be looking at the physical differences some of them have compared to others. You will have to understand the environment each of them needs to thrive as well. That will narrow your decision down to at least a few, as you might not want to invest in a lot of new equipment just yet.

Something we will also discuss is the potency differences between some of the strains. While you might be looking to cultivate something mellow for meditation, someone else wants to use them for a life-changing trip or ego death. It is always good to consider everything before getting into it all at once. Otherwise, you might end up regretting your choice to pursue magic mushroom cultivation.

What to Expect

There are a few differences to be observed between the most popular strains for cultivation. Let's quickly go over the basics before delving into the different strains themselves. Here we will construct a list of a few things to consider when deciding on what type of magic mushroom and/or experience you are looking for.

Spore Availability

Firstly, you will have to start looking at what species are readily available in your area. If you have some friends with previous psilocybin experience, you can ask them if they know. If they do not, you can always ask them if they know anyone who might have some experience or who might even cultivate their own. It is always a good idea to gather as much information as possible.

If you cannot find anyone to help you out, the internet is your new friend!

You can find online stores or forums to help you out with finding the available species in your area. While going over a few popular species, I will try to narrow the areas down for you as best I can.

That way, you can start right off the bat with cultivation.

Natural Availability

Something you can consider when looking for spores or your next experience is where you might be able to find naturally occurring psilocybin mushrooms. There is always the option to go out in search of psilocybin mushrooms; however, it might be more dangerous than you realize.

Firstly, your experience out in the wild may be lacking, so going out to remote areas you are not used to can be very irresponsible. Secondly, if you are not an experienced mycologist, there is a very big chance of misidentifying the species of mushroom. In short, you might end up poisoning yourself. However, if you find someone experienced enough to help you or if you feel you are experienced enough yourself, it can be an option. You will be able to find many species in the wild if you know where to look. When going over the popular species, I will try to outline where they are the most abundant in nature.

You will be able to take spores from them as well, which can save you a bit of money on cultivation. Later in the book, there will be a guide on harvesting the spores as well, be it from your own cultivated mushrooms or ones you found.

I do not recommend foraging for psilocybin mushrooms as your first option, due to the possible dangers it may present.

Cultivability

You will have to be sure the strain you want to cultivate is not too picky when it comes to its environment. Later, when we go over the difference in strains, you will realize that most psilocybin mushrooms prefer almost the same environments for growth.

However, the specific one you might be looking to grow can prefer a warmer, damper, dryer, or colder environment than what you are currently living in. In that case, you will have to start thinking about building a properly controlled habitat for your mushrooms. Not to worry, however, we will be going over those advanced growing habitats as well. It's just something for you to start considering, or at least know about.

Something else to look out for when deciding on the cultivation of a specific strain will be the actual yield. Some strains will yield a big amount per harvest, which can be around 70 grams when dried. Other strains might yield less, due to the difference in the physical size of the fruiting bodies. The number of magic mushrooms per harvest can be a deciding factor in your choice of strain.

Potency

The potency surrounding any strain of psilocybin mushroom is still very debatable. Some believe the difference in potency is so little that ultimately it doesn't matter. I can tell you out of my own personal experience, however, that it does.

Others will say that the amount of psilocybin found in each fruiting body will be different from another. While this might be true, the overall difference in each body will be very slight, if you cultivate them properly. When one part gets more nutrients than the other, then there will obviously be a difference.

The potency of each strain does not necessarily refer to just the amount of psilocybin in each fruiting body, however. The overall experience can differ between strains through simple means. Some might provide you with more visuals, while others can provide you with more of a hallucinogenic experience.

When discussing the strains, I will highlight for you the exact experience one might have when consuming each.

Uses

While on the topic of potency, we can discuss the difference in uses as well. The potency and experience of each strain will determine the use for each of them. When we look at the different personal uses, we can narrow them down to a few for now.

Recreational - When using magic mushrooms for recreational use, you might want to decide on a strain that will be less harsh on your digestive system. Some strains can cause a bit of gas when consumed, depending on the person. When cultivating for recreational use, you will most likely want a strain with higher potency as well. There are a few strains that have a stronger taste as well, so if you are going to consume big amounts, that might change the strain you will want to cultivate.

Medicinal - This might be a more controversial topic, as not everyone understands the medicinal value behind mushrooms, especially psilocybin ones. Even when you do understand the possible benefits for your condition, you are not necessarily qualified to diagnose that condition or assign treatment.

Research in this field is also minimal at the moment. Most of it covers psychological and emotional help. The only confirmed physical benefits from its use are for addiction, as we discussed previously. If you believe you might benefit from psilocybin mushrooms in such a way, who am I to stop you? I would suggest, however, discussing it with a medical professional first.

Spiritual - A spiritual journey is something I feel everyone should embark on. While some might have a longer journey than others, it doesn't mean that it is of less value.

Many find the use of psilocybin a must on your spiritual journey. If you are looking for mushrooms to help in regard to that, then you will have to decide carefully on the strain you want to cultivate. A spiritual journey can be scary, straight-up terrifying in some cases. Existential dread can sometimes cripple us during our journeys. The use of a very potent strain might increase that feeling, leaving you terrified. A more mellow strain will help you deal with that dread, easing you through your journey.

That is why the ancient tribes used these substances in their ceremonies. The effects will help you transcend your spiritual journey.

I will be pointing out what strains are best for a spiritual journey, so not to worry.

Psychological and Emotional - Some of you might be looking to treat your emotional or psychological conditions with magic mushrooms. While there is nothing inherently wrong with that, you will have to be careful. Using the wrong strain or dosage can actually make everything worse.

When looking into cultivating these mushrooms for psychological or emotional treatment, I would suggest speaking with a professional mental health representative first.

If you do feel that an experience from magic mushroom consumption helped you in some way, and you wish to repeat that experience, I will not stop you. Many people who feel depressed, experience anxiety, have a lack of focus, or lack motivation may find that magic mushrooms can be quite beneficial, so if that is you, go for it.

I will label which strains might assist you in the specific treatment you are looking for as best I can.

Individual Experience

Ultimately, you will have to make a decision yourself. I will not be able to decide for you what type of strain you will want to cultivate. I stated previously that you might want to try magic mushrooms first before deciding to cultivate them. That still applies now. When deciding on the strain you wish to cultivate, it is a good idea to actually experience the effects each can provide.

Now, this might be difficult, considering the legality of magic mushrooms around the world. However, the more experience you gain, the more informed of a decision you will be able to make.

You see the thing is, some individuals might have a completely different experience from what you had, on the same strain. The best you can do is at least narrow down your reaction to as many strains as possible. While a list of strains and their effects will give you a guideline, personal experience is the best way that you will be able to confirm what works for you.

I remember I ate some shrooms with my partner one night; it was her first time trying it. She ended up laughing for two hours straight, I'm not even exaggerating. By the end of the night, she was in pain due to all the laughter—she could not even walk! I, on the other hand, was completely fine and only had mild hallucinations.

Now you can see what the importance is of actually deciding on a strain to cultivate. In the end, magic mushrooms will be able to give you the experience that you are looking for. Some strains might be slightly off from what you expected, but that is how you will learn.

Psychoactive Mushroom Species

Here you will be able to have a look at a few of the popular psilocybin mushrooms species out there. Keep in mind these are not the only ones available. They will, however, be the ones you are most likely to find in nature or in shops online. Some of them have different variants, but they are of the same species and so they retain most of the same effects.

Potency levels for reference:

1. Relaxed
2. Mellow
3. High
4. Very High
5. Extremely High
6. Toxic

Cultivation difficulty level for reference:

1. Easy
2. Moderate
3. Difficult
4. Near Impossible

Amanita muscaria

The first on this list is not actually a psilocybin-containing mushroom. It is, however, very well known as a psychoactive mushroom. This mushroom has long been seen as one of the most important mushrooms for mankind.

Many know it by the names fly agaric or fly amanita.

The reason I am placing this one on the list is simply due to the significant role it has played throughout history.

PSILOCYBIN MUSHROOMS

This mushroom has long been the central ingredient for potions and brews in ancient tribal and religious ceremonies, especially in Siberian, American, and European rituals. This mushroom has also been implicated in the Eleusinian Mysteries of the ancient Greek pilgrimage to Eleusis.

Potency level: Varies between very high and toxic

Cultivation difficulty: Near impossible

To follow are the scientific classifications of *A. muscaria*:

Domain:	Eukarya
Kingdom:	Fungi
Phylum:	Basidiomycota
Class:	Agaricomycetes
Order:	Agaricales
Family:	Amanitaceae
Genus:	Amanita
Species:	*A. muscaria*

This mushroom is quite difficult to cultivate for personal use, and many do not recommend it. *A. muscaria* has an almost symbiotic relationship with the roots of a tree, making it very difficult to cultivate indoors.

The mycelia dig into and live inside the roots of mostly pine trees, gathering nutrients from the tree and soil. While it is possible to try and cultivate *A. muscaria* in your backyard, many have tried and failed. Not to mention that it can end up too toxic for consumption.

PSILOCYBIN MUSHROOMS

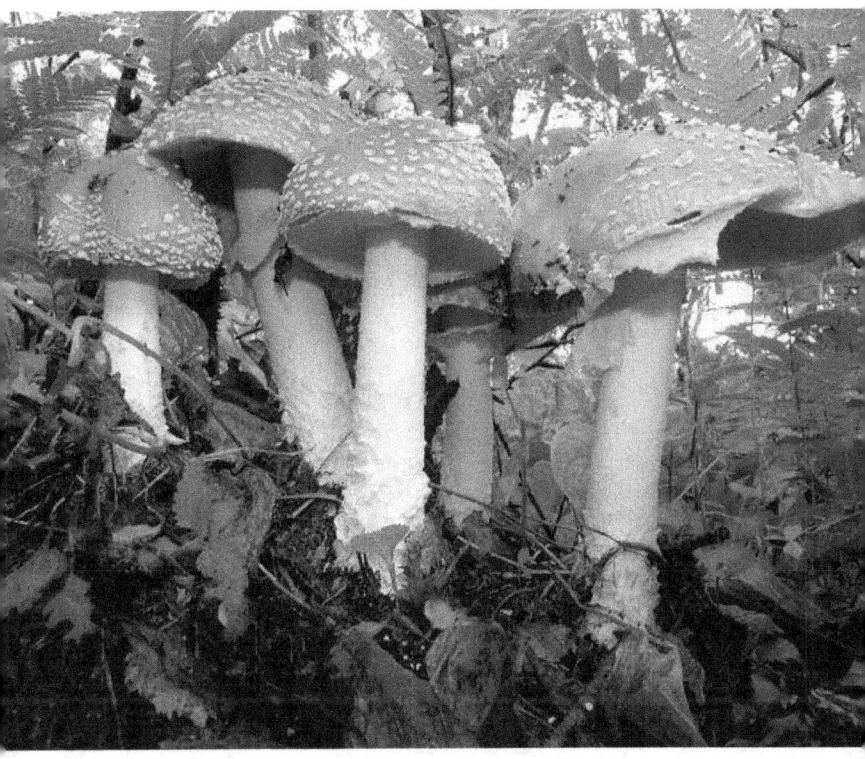

It has the most identifiable morphology compared to the others on this list. It sports a bright red or orange cap with white spots and white gills. It can grow to around 7 inches across and almost 11 inches tall. Many people credit it to be the tastiest as well, having a mildly sweet flavor with a savory scent.

You can try to cultivate this one entirely at your own risk.

Psilocybe allenii

This one is quite new to the family of psilocybin mushrooms, being scientifically identified only in 2012 as its own species. It was known in San Francisco as an unidentified *Psilocybe cyanescens* variant for a few years before being officially classified.

Potency level: Very high

Cultivation difficulty: Difficult

To follow are the scientific classifications of *P. allenii*:

Domain: Eukarya
Kingdom: Fungi
Phylum: Basidiomycota
Class: Agaricomycetes
Order: Agaricales
Family: Hymenogastraceae
Genus: Psilocybe
Species: *P. allenii*

PSILOCYBIN MUSHROOMS

This species can be found naturally occurring in the northwestern parts of America. Cultivation of this species is not too difficult; however, it can become problematic. *P. allenii* has a tendency to only grow from rotten wood or the wood chips used for landscaping. A specialized substrate will be required.

These mushrooms can vary in shape quite a lot depending on the nutrients absorbed. Its cap can grow up to 1.7 inches across with a convex or bell-shaped cap. The stem can be up to 2.3 inches long with a thickness of about 0.1 inches. The cap color is usually brown to a fading yellow-brown with cinnamon-brown gills. The stem is milky white with bluish bruising.

PSILOCYBIN MUSHROOMS

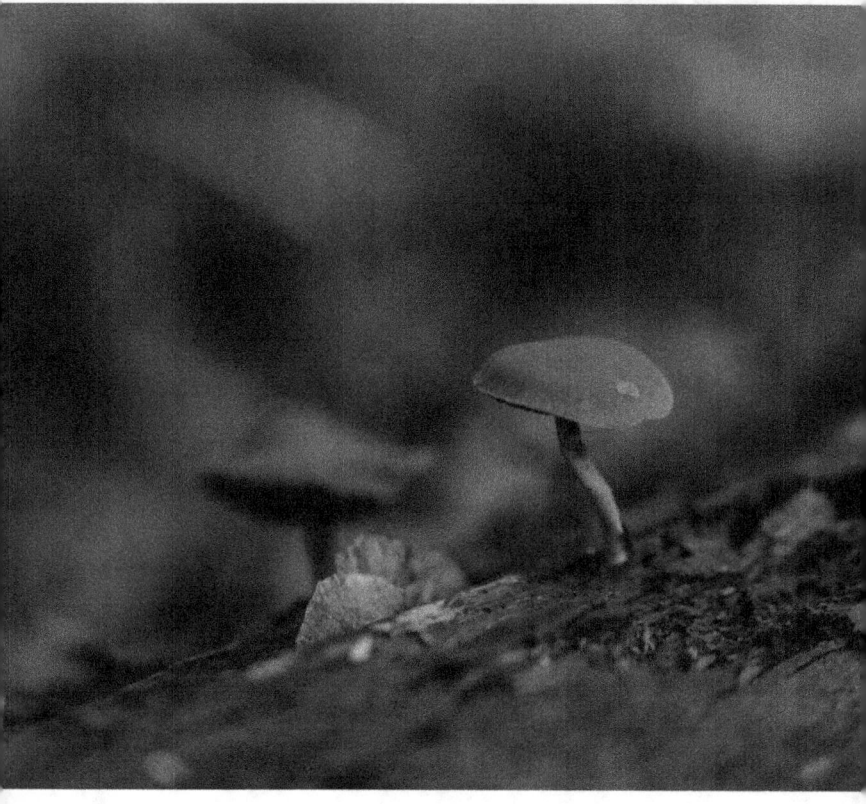

PSILOCYBIN MUSHROOMS

This particular species has a known effect called wood-lovers paralysis (WLP).

Psilocybin mushrooms that exclusively grow from wood cause this. It can lead to the user quite literally being paralyzed for anything between a few minutes to a few hours. There have been reports from people who have either lost all footing, with their legs buckling under them when walking. There have also been incidents of uncontrollable urination due to the paralysis.

Inexperienced cultivators might want to try something else.

Psilocybe azurescens

This small mushroom can be found naturally growing in western parts of Oregon and California. It was first discovered by Boy Scouts out camping near the Columbia River in Oregon.

Potency level: Extremely High

Cultivation difficulty: Difficult

To follow are the scientific classifications of *P. azurescens*:

Domain:	Eukarya
Kingdom:	Fungi
Phylum:	Basidiomycota
Class:	Agaricomycetes
Order:	Agaricales

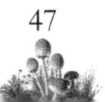

PSILOCYBIN MUSHROOMS

Family: Hymenogastraceae
Genus: Psilocybe
Species: *P. azurescens*

Cultivation of this species can be quite easy; however, it also has a tendency to only grow from rotten wood or wood chips and favors colder temperatures. Cultivating this one will require a specialized substrate.

Consumption of this strain may also lead to wood-lovers paralysis (WLP).

The appearance of this little mushroom does not vary much. They are usually found to be between 1–3 inches across, although they are usually on the smaller side. The cap is conic to convex, which will expand and flatten out with age. They rarely grow to about 7 inches but it does happen; they have silky-white stems. The gills are brown with white edges.

This strain is quite potent; you can expect to experience intense visuals even with smaller doses. The average amount of psilocybin per mushroom in other species is usually 0.10% to 0.50%. The amount in *P. azurescens* is 1.60% to 1.80%, which gives you an idea of exactly how potent they are.

P. azurescens is not the best option for a first-time cultivator, but not the worst either.

PSILOCYBIN MUSHROOMS

Psilocybe caerulescens

Known as the "landslide" mushroom by many due to its Spanish name "derrumbe," it is theorized to have been used by Aztec shamans and is currently being used by Mazatec shamans. Many people compare the taste of this mushroom to the taste of cucumber.

Potency level: High

Cultivation difficulty: Moderate

To follow are the scientific classifications of *P. caerulescens*:

Domain:	Eukarya
Kingdom:	Fungi
Phylum:	Basidiomycota
Class:	Agaricomycetes
Order:	Agaricales
Family:	Strophariaceae
Genus:	Psilocybe
Species:	*P. caerulescens*

This mushroom can be found in southeastern America, with the first reported sightings in Alabama. It can be found growing from soil or even lawns, usually away from direct sunlight.

Cultivation of this species is fairly easy, as it does not need a specialized substrate. Many prefer using rye grain, as the yield of a harvest is usually bigger; however, any other substrate can be used.

The cap is usually found to be about 3–5 inches across and 3–5 inches long. The stem is a reddish white, measuring around 0.4 inches thick. The color of the cap is usually a yellowish brown or straw yellow. The gills are dark brown.

The effects of this mushroom are not as intense as others, so it is usually recommended for beginners. The combination of easy cultivation and level of potency makes it a good candidate for first-time cultivators.

Psilocybe caerulipes

This mushroom is quite rare in the wild and is known as "blue-foot." It will grow in very solitary and dense forest areas, usually sprouting from wood debris and plant matter. *P. caerulipes* was first found in eastern North America, between Ontario and North Carolina; however, it has recently been found as far south as Mexico.

Potency level: High

Cultivation difficulty: Difficult

To follow are the scientific classifications of *P. caerulipes*:

Domain:	Eukarya
Kingdom:	Fungi
Phylum:	Basidiomycota
Class:	Agaricomycetes
Order:	Agaricales
Family:	Hymenogastraceae
Genus:	Psilocybe
Species:	*P. caerulipes*

The appearance of this mushroom is quite unique, hence the name blue-foot. The base of the stem will usually have a blue hue to it, with the cap having more of a brownish-green tint. The cap is not too large, only growing about 1.1 inches across, shaped convexed to flattened. It can grow to about 2.5 inches long, with very dense light-brown gills.

Due to *P. caerulipes* feeding off dead wood, WLP is a very likely effect of consumption. Laughter and a surge of emotions are also among common effects of this species.

Cultivation can prove to be quite difficult, given the rarity of spores. Even when spores are acquired, the substrate will have to be specialized, containing some wood debris. Some claim that indoor cultivation is impossible, with outdoor cultivation being the best option, or a highly advanced indoor regulation system is needed.

This species is not recommended for first-time cultivators.

Psilocybe cubensis

Being one of the most popular options for both first-time cultivators and first-time users, *P. cubensis* is very well known, and spores are abundant. Certain strains include Golden Teachers and Blue-Meanies. This specific species is also known for its uses in spiritual healing rituals and microdosing.

Potency level: Relaxed to high depending on cultivation method

Cultivation difficulty: Easy

PSILOCYBIN MUSHROOMS

To follow are the scientific classifications of *P. cubensis*:

Domain: Eukarya
Kingdom: Fungi
Phylum: Basidiomycota
Class: Agaricomycetes
Order: Agaricales
Family: Hymenogastraceae
Genus:
Species:

This mushroom is abundant throughout America and is quite easily identifiable. The cap is usually between 1–3 inches across with a coned tip and convex edge. The gills are wider in the center with a greyish color to them. It can grow to about 10 inches in length, with the stem staying fairly thin, about 0.5 inches thick. The stem is a yellowing-white color.

The substrate required to cultivate this mushroom does not have to be specialized. It grows naturally in tropical environments, favoring cattle pastures for the manure. Humidity requirements can sometimes be a bit higher than others but not so much that specialized equipment is needed.

Effects felt when consuming *P. cubensis* are usually mild depending on the dosage. An introspective and relaxed experience is usual for this strain.

Cultivation for first timers is highly recommended.

PSILOCYBIN MUSHROOMS

Psilocybe cyanescens

Known as the "wavy-cap" mushroom, this species is one of varied potency compared to others. *P. cyanescens* is found to be rather bitter compared to other species, which makes consuming them raw quite nauseating. It can mainly be found in the northwest coastal area, going down south as far as San Francisco. It is also the most common species in the northwest.

Potency level: High to extremely high

Cultivation Difficulty: Moderate

To follow are the scientific classifications of *P. cyanescens*:

Domain:	Eukarya
Kingdom:	Fungi
Phylum:	Basidiomycota
Class:	Agaricomycetes
Order:	Agaricales
Family:	Hymenogastraceae
Genus:	Psilocybe
Species:	*P. caerulipes*

The wavy cap of this species can grow to around 1.7 inches across with a convex wavey cap. The stem itself will grow to only about 2.3 inches. The color will vary between brown and yellow-brown for the cap and a smooth silky white for the stem. The gills are usually a dark greyish brown.

Wood chips are primarily used when cultivating this mushroom, so WLP is very likely when consumed. The WLP effect is less intense than with other wood-loving species, however. It is seen as the easier wood-loving species to cultivate, so it does make a good choice for someone looking to get into wood-loving mushroom cultivation.

P. cyanescens is one of the few mushrooms to contain psilocybin and baeocystin, which makes the experience quite unique, explained by some as a "rollercoaster ride." For comparison, 2 grams of dried *P. cyanescens* is just as potent, if not more so, than 5 grams of dried *P. cubensis*. Many people suggest taking a gram less with this species than you usually would with others.

Recommended for cultivators getting into wood-loving mushrooms.

Psilocybe mexicana

This mushroom was used extensively more than 2,000 years ago by Aztecs in spiritual rituals and was known to them as "god fungus." It grows at higher elevations and is very rarely seen in lower elevations. It can be found more to the south of Mexico, on to Costa Rica, and Guatemala.

Potency level: Mellow to high

Cultivation difficulty: Moderate

To follow are the scientific classifications of *P. mexicana*:

PSILOCYBIN MUSHROOMS

Domain: Eukarya
Kingdom: Fungi
Phylum: Basidiomycota
Class: Agaricomycetes
Order: Agaricales
Family: Hymenogastraceae
Genus: Psilocybe
Species: *P. caerulipes*

P. mexicana is well known for its umbrella-like appearance, so identification is fairly easy. The cap will grow to about 1.1 inches across with the shape of a halfway-opened umbrella. The stem can grow to about 5 inches tall, but it is usually very thin at 0.1 inches. The color of the cap is a straw-brown or beige color, the gills are a purple-brown, and the stem is a reddish brown.

PSILOCYBIN MUSHROOMS

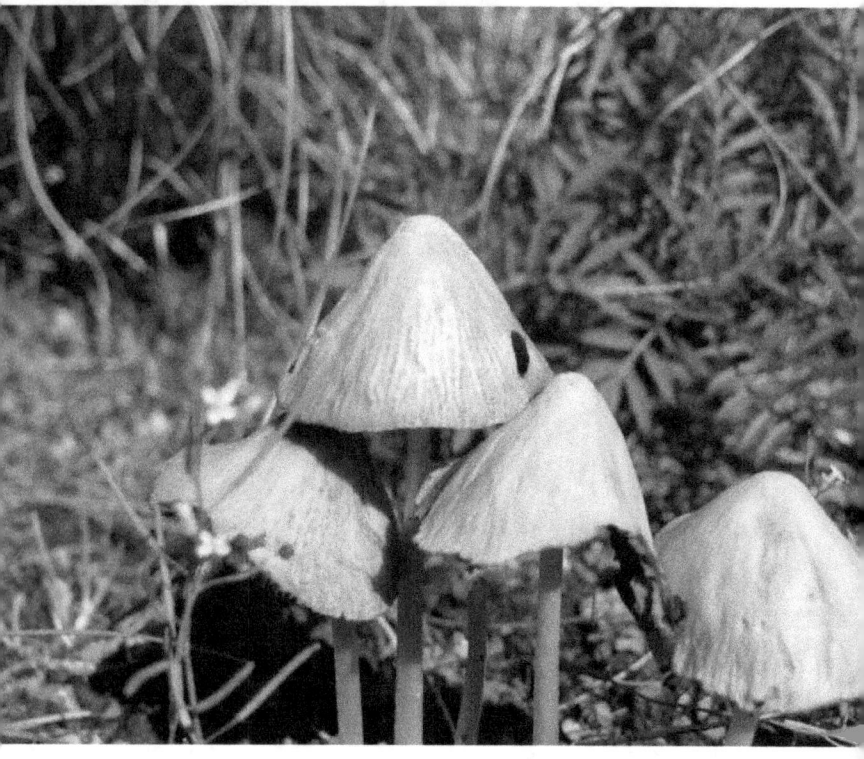

Cultivation of this strain is seen as low maintenance by many who have previous experience. They can, however, have difficulty fruiting when not cultivated at the correct elevation, so the suggested elevation is around 980–1,800 ft above sea level.

As for the experience itself, it is usually described as light and happy, accompanied by mild visuals depending on the dosage. Many people use this species for the treatment of cancer patients with depression, or spiritual awakenings.

Cultivation is not recommended for someone below the suggested elevation.

Psilocybe semilanceata

This mushroom is known as a "liberty cap" and is one of the most potent species found in nature. It is sometimes said to be the most popular magic mushroom in the world, but that is debatable. This little mushroom was classified as far back as the 19th century.

Potency level: Very high to extremely high

Cultivation difficulty: Difficult

To follow are the scientific classifications of *P. Semilanceata*:

Domain:	Eukarya
Kingdom:	Fungi
Phylum:	Basidiomycota
Class:	Agaricomycetes

PSILOCYBIN MUSHROOMS

Order: Agaricales
Family: Hymenogastraceae
Genus: Psilocybe
Species: *P. caerulipes*

This species will grow in grasslands all over America. While *P. cubensis* will use cow dung for nutrients, *P. Semilanceata* feeds on the roots of the grass. It prefers a lower temperature, but cultivation is not made difficult by this.

P. Semilanceata also resembles the shape of an umbrella, but with a few noticeable differences from *P. mexicana*. The cap will only grow out to just about 1 inch across and 4 inches long. The shape will be cone-like, similar to a halfway-opened umbrella.

The stem will, however, have a slight curve in the center as it grows out, almost like a zigzag. The cap is quite varied but will usually resemble either a chestnut-brown to a yellow-brown tan. The stem is white-brown with a darker brown towards the base, and the gills are grey with purple-brown edges.

The effects felt by this mushroom are similar to those felt after the consumption of LSD. A heavy distortion of color and depth in vision will be experienced; some users have reported slight nausea, however.

This strain is not recommended for first-time cultivators.

PSILOCYBIN MUSHROOMS

Psilocybe stuntzii

This species is often confused for the *Galerina marginata* fungus, which is a highly toxic mushroom. Many poisonings by fungus have been attributed to this confusion.

P. stuntzii is also known as Stunt's Blue Legs—named after a mycologist who studied it, David Stunts—or Blue Ringers. It can be found throughout the Northwest and favors soils rich in bark mulch and wood chips.

Potency level: Mellow

Cultivation difficulty: Moderate

To follow are the scientific classifications of *P. stuntzii*:

Domain: Eukarya
Kingdom: Fungi
Phylum: Basidiomycota
Class: Agaricomycetes
Order: Agaricales
Family: Hymenogastraceae
Genus: Psilocybe
Species: *P. caerulipes*

P. stuntzii is known to have an almost slimy looking cap, growing to about 1.3 inches across. The shape is convex to almost flat. Growing to around 3 inches in height, the stem is 0.5 inches thick but will expand around the base. The gills are violet-brown with the cap being a slight greenish brown. The stem is silky white.

Cultivation has been found to be easier in the Northwest, growing naturally all year around Washington. Due to its need for wood and mulch, it is easier to cultivate outdoors around the edges of wooden buildings or trees.

The effects felt by this species are usually in the range of increased heart rate, bursts of energy, and light visuals. It is not recommended for users with any form of cardiovascular problems.

Cultivation is recommended over foraging, due to the confusion with *Galerina marginata*, although beginners might have difficulty cultivating it.

Psilocybe tampanensis

P. tampanensis is a very rare species that was once found in Florida, but not since. It was found again years later in Mississippi, but its habitat preferences are not exactly known.

Potency level: Mellow to high

Cultivation difficulty: Moderate

To follow are the scientific classifications of *P. tampanensis*:

Domain:	Eukarya
Kingdom:	Fungi
Phylum:	Basidiomycota
Class:	Agaricomycetes
Order:	Agaricales

PSILOCYBIN MUSHROOMS

Family: Hymenogastraceae
Genus: Psilocybe
Species: *P. caerulipes*

While it might be rare, it is not difficult to get a hold of the spores themselves. Cultivation is not exactly difficult either; however, more patience is required as the colonization speed is slower than other species.

The caps of this species are usually convex, with the edges flaring up slightly. They can grow to about 0.9 inches across and the stems to about 4 inches long. The caps are very smooth with a straw-brown color in the center and straw-yellow on the edges. The stems are white-yellow with the gills being purple-brown.

The effects felt from this species usually include heightened senses and vibrant visuals.

P. tampanensis is not recommended to first-time cultivators, due to the limited amount of information available for them. If you are able to get your hands on the spores, however, you can give it a try.

Have You Decided?

When looking at all the different species available for cultivation, it can be a bit overwhelming at first.

Can I give you some advice?

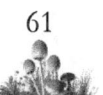

Start out with a species that is easy to cultivate. Some people decide to go for a moderate one due to the high potency and end up getting discouraged when it doesn't work out. You can always try again in the future, but when that first time actually works out, the boost in confidence will help in cultivating a more difficult strain later on.

You do not necessarily need highly potent shrooms for the first try; you can always buy some somewhere. The idea is to get used to the process of cultivation first.

Have you decided? Let's get to cultivating!

PSILOCYBIN MUSHROOMS

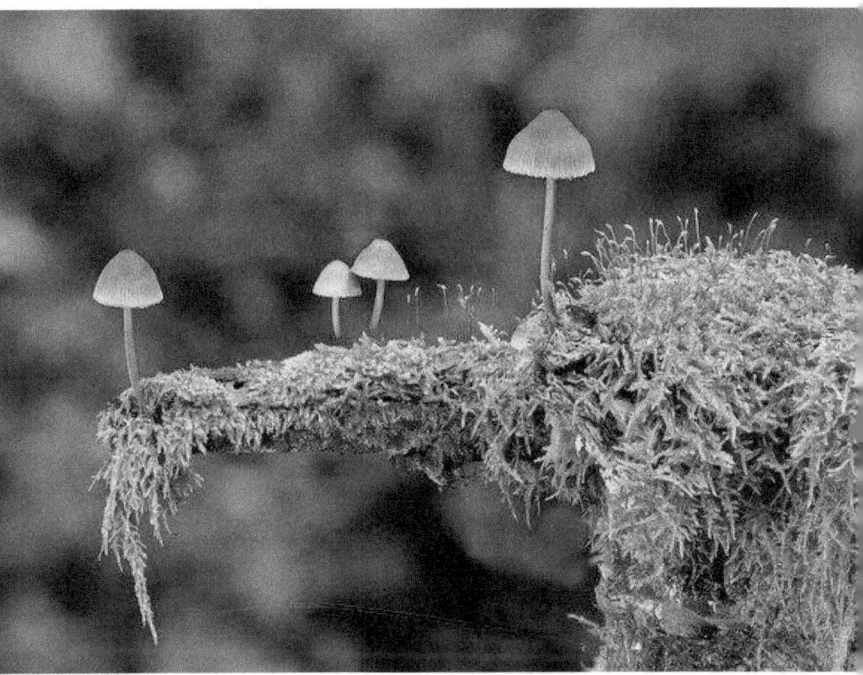

CHAPTER 3

CULTIVATING PSILOCYBIN MUSHROOMS

Cultivating mushrooms can be quite a daunting task; nevertheless, it can be done. You most likely understand the possible benefits of psilocybin mushrooms by now, and you have most likely decided on a species to focus on.

Next will be deciding on the method of cultivation.

Where to Grow

While many people are familiar with a few ways of cultivating mushrooms, some people do not know that you can actually grow mushrooms either in a controlled environment or outside.

One of the first steps in your journey will begin with the decision of where you are actually going to start the process of cultivation. This will all depend on the species of mushroom you have decided on. Some of them might be easier to cultivate outdoors, where others will only be possible to do indoors.

Firstly, let's get one of the main issues for cultivation out of the way. The cultivation, possession, and consumption of magic mushrooms are illegal in most countries, including the United States. While there are some states that have decriminalized it, you will have to look up some of the laws and restrictions in your area surrounding magic mushrooms.

Okay, now you can decide on where to grow your goodies.

Outside

When it comes to outdoor psilocybin mushroom cultivation, some people are a bit misinformed. While it is possible, many prefer cultivating their mushrooms indoors, as the process is much easier to regulate.

There are a few kits out there that you can buy specifically made with outdoor cultivation in mind. These usually include a specific species of mushrooms with a specialized substrate. If you are looking to go the outdoor way, then you might want to decide on a wood-loving species of mushroom. Most of the premade kits out there usually come inoculated with *Psilocybe azurescens* mycelium. That makes it easy as you completely skip the inoculation process.

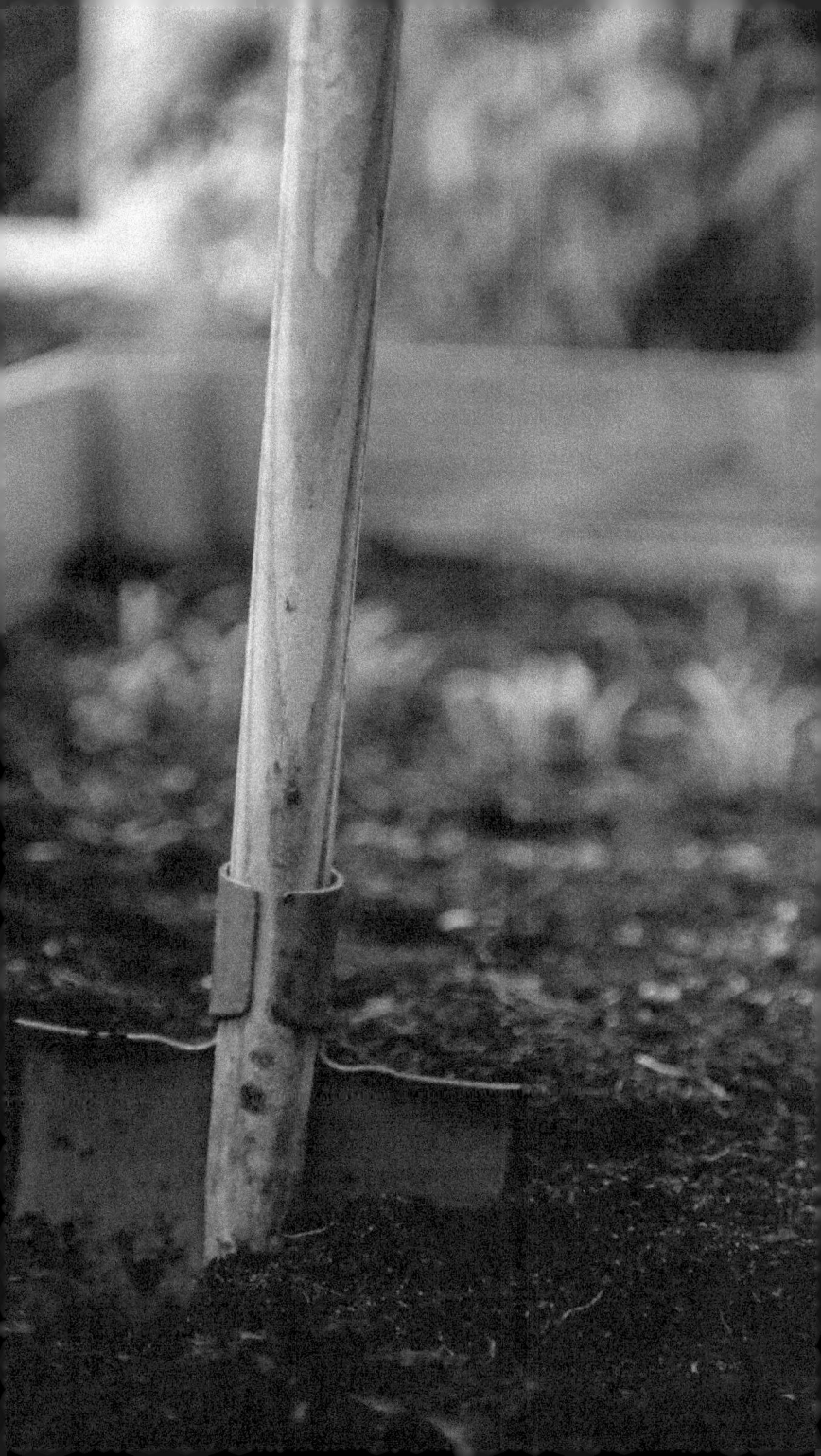

You do run quite a few risks when going the outdoors route, which is why I do not usually recommend this method to first timers or beginners. The biggest risk will be from the contamination of your growth patch. Seeing as this is the outdoors, you do not necessarily know if there are any other mycelium networks running through your soil. Even when you use a pot or container outdoors, the chance of contamination through natural spore dispersal is also a high risk.

What happens when your patch gets contaminated? Worst-case scenario is that your mushrooms will become poisonous, you consume them, and you end up in the hospital. The best-case scenario is that you lose the batch and will have to start over. While there are ways to reduce the risk of contamination, it is very difficult for beginners.

I will be going over the steps of outdoors cultivation, however, so if you have already decided on an outdoor location, not to worry! For now, we are just going through your options.

Indoors

Growing magic mushrooms indoors is by far the easiest method of cultivation. When I say the easiest method, I do not necessarily mean it is easy overall. Cultivating mushrooms takes time, effort, supplies, and patience, and you will need to be tentative.

The mistake many first growers make is not taking it seriously enough. They usually end up with a contaminated first batch or a batch devoid of fruiting bodies.

When deciding on a species for indoor cultivation, there are quite a few options. The only ones you might have difficulty with are the wood-loving species. While it is not impossible to cultivate them indoors, you will need specialized substrates and extra care.

Something else to consider when growing indoors is also the method with which you will be doing so. There are quite a few methods that we will be going over momentarily. Many beginners prefer a simple jar and cake method, while others prefer a method with a larger yield. We will be going over all the available methods, so not to worry. It is just a good thing to know you have at least a few different options.

There are quite a few kits available online as well. We will be focusing on the basics of each, as well as how to do it all by yourself from scratch.

Getting Started

Okay, I know you are very excited to start the cultivation process, and we are almost there. It's just that there are a few keywords and terms I want to go over with you so that you do not get lost on a technical term or cultivation jargon. Some of the words or terms I have already used in

PSILOCYBIN MUSHROOMS

previous chapters. If you got lost on them, not to worry; I will outline the meaning of them here.

In the first chapter, you had a brief look at the life cycle of the fungus known as magic mushrooms. Just in case you forgot, here is the basic life cycle:

Spores - Germination - Mycelium Network - Pins - Stems - Fruiting bodies - Spores

Terminology

To follow is a list of technical terms and words we will be using throughout the cultivation process:

- **Colonization** - This is the phase mycelium enters when it is starting to grow throughout the substrate. You will hit this phase after the inoculation of your substrate.

- **Cake** - This is a term used for when a substrate has fused together with mycelium. This usually happens in jars or tubs as the whole mass becomes a hard substance resembling a cake.

- **Fruiting Body** - This is the big part of the mushroom at the top. Most of the psilocybin is contained within the fruiting bodies. When you start seeing them, you are nearly finished.

- **Fruiting Chamber** - Depending on your method of cultivation, the term fruiting chamber will refer to the container being used in order to actually grow the mushrooms. We will go into detail regarding the best fruiting chambers for each method later on.

- **Germination** - This term is used in order to refer to the process of a spore first starting its formations connecting and growing, becoming mycelium.

- **Inoculation** - This is the part where you introduce your spores to whichever substrate you decided on. The method of inoculation will be different depending on the substrate, method of cultivation, and spores. Not to worry, though, we will go over the processes of inoculation for each of them.

- **Mycelium** - As we discussed in the first chapter, mycelium is the vegetative state of fungi. When you see it grow, it means you are on the right track.

- **Spores** - Almost everyone interested in mushroom cultivation of any kind will know what spores are. If you do not, however, not to worry! Here is a quick breakdown of what a spore is. A spore is a unit of sexual or asexual reproduction in biology for fungi. Spores are forcefully ejected by a fungus for what can essentially be called reproduction. Basically, you will need some if you want to grow mushrooms.

- **Spore Print** - This is a method of gathering spores. A print is made by using sterile card stock, foil, plastic, or any flat surface, and then basically pressing it up against the gills of a mushroom. A print containing spores will then be left on the surface.

- **Spore Syringe** - This is something you can usually get from online stores. It is technically not illegal to sell spores of any kind, so it is safe to buy them. These syringes are filled with a special type of liquid in order to contain and preserve the spores of the requested species.

- **Substrate** - This will basically be the food for your magic mushroom. Different species enjoy different types of substrate. Most species will be able to grow in any substrate; however, there are some that require specific nutrients, like wood-loving species. Depending on the species, they will grow bigger or stay small if their favorite substrate is not used. Common substrates may include rice, straw, types of grain, compost, mulch, manure, woodchips, and even birdseed. A mixture of them can be used as well.

- **TEK** - This is an abbreviation used in the mushroom cultivation community for technique. You will see the use of PF-TEK a lot online, for example. It is short for Psilocybe Fanaticus

Technique, a theory for home growing off which many other methods are based.

- **Sterilization** - This is when you make sure there are no bacterial or fungal contaminants. You will be doing a lot of sterilization while cultivating mushrooms; otherwise, you will end up with contaminated magic mushrooms. Sterilization is done with rubbing alcohol, steam, fire, or a disinfectant like Lysol. It will all depend on the method of cultivation, but be prepared to have and/or use one or all of those items.

- **Veil** - This is a part of the mushroom that will play an important role when harvesting your mushrooms after the fruiting process. It connects the edge of the cap of the mushroom to the stem. This ensures the gills containing the spores are protected. The veil tears, later on, exposing the gills.

These terms will be used in this book, and they are used all over the internet when you search for information regarding mushroom cultivation. It is a good idea to make sure you understand them all.

Cultivation Methods and Substrates

There are numerous ways one can try to grow magic mushrooms. You will have to decide on a method before continuing your journey. Once you decide on a method, you can pick a substrate. The same goes for already having a substrate in mind that might be more accessible to you. Then you can decide on a method more suited to your substrate.

You will have to get your hands on some equipment no matter what method you choose, but you most likely knew that already.

Something to also think about is the actual time it will take for the whole process. Not to worry, as the complete process from start to finish usually doesn't take more than 4–6 weeks.

Cultivation methods can be broken up into a few categories, so let's start with the first.

Pick a Substrate

Okay, if you already have a substrate in mind, you can skip to selecting a fruiting chamber. It is a good idea, however, to make sure you understand how your substrate and other substrates can make a difference in cultivation. Let's go over the best substrate options and the methods best suited to them. Keep in mind you will have a substrate, which you inoculate. You will then have a bulk substrate which you will mix in later on so the mushrooms can get more nutrients.

Many people still do not understand the difference between using a method containing grain spawn or perhaps something like the PF-TEK. Well, let's make sure you are not one of them.

Grain Spawn

Grain spawn is used when you want to be able to spread your mycelium around a container, like a mono-tub. This makes it quite an easy choice for someone who wants to yield a bigger batch, but it does have a few drawbacks.

When you use grain spawn, you will have to either find a form of grain that was sterilized properly, or you will have to sterilize it yourself. Many stores and online shops do sell sterilized and sealed grain packs.

If you are looking to use grain spawn, which is what I used for my first cultivation experience, you will have to decide on buying a sterile and sealed pack or sterilizing your own.

PSILOCYBIN MUSHROOMS

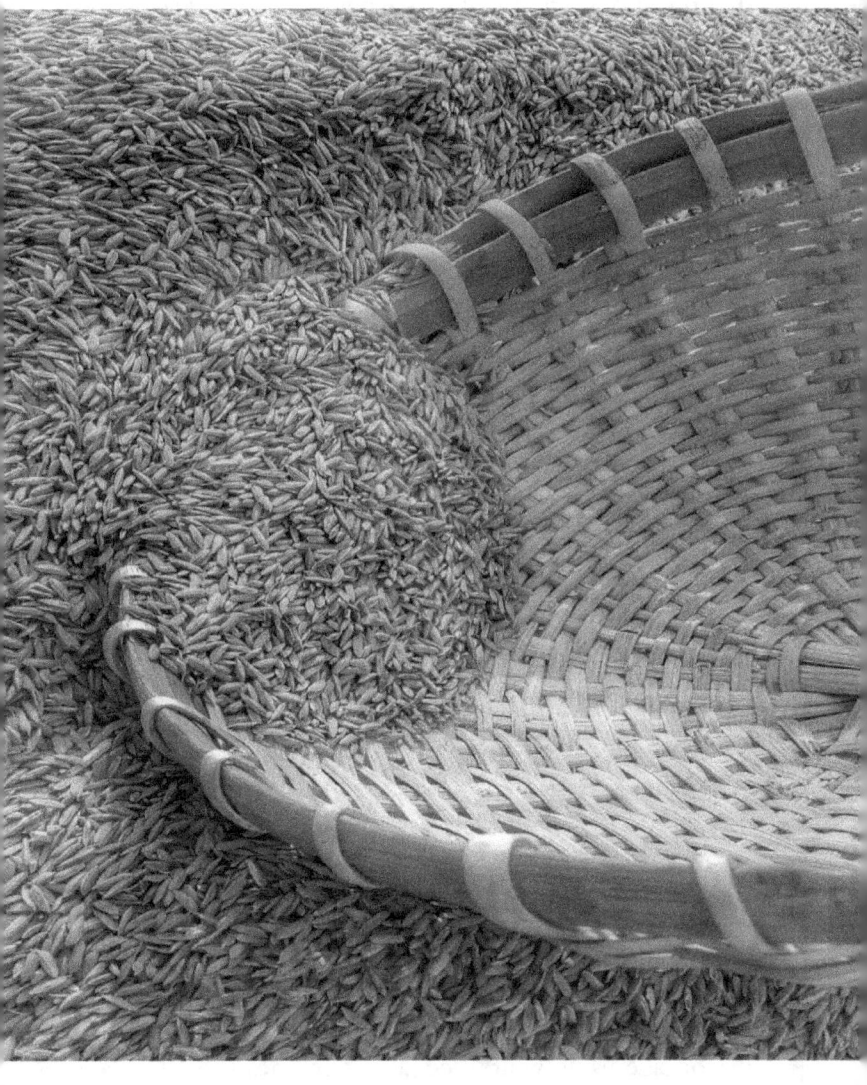

Buying a sterile pack is the easiest by far and will require less effort on your side. The one drawback, however, is that the shops will not always have the grain available that you are looking for. Presterilized packs are best suited for spore syringes, as most of them come with a self-healing injection port.

If you decide on getting your own grain and sterilizing it yourself, do not worry. I will be going over the sterilization process as well. All that is left is to choose what type of grain you will want to use.

Rye - Many suggest rye grain as a first choice, due to the fact that it holds in moisture better than other grains. It is, however, difficult to find in small amounts and can be quite expensive. I do not suggest it for a first-time grower, especially if you are only growing a small amount.

Wheat berries - Wheat grain and seeds are known as wheat berries and are the next best choice. They can be sterilized using the same method as rye grain, and they perform almost on the same level when it comes to the yield.

Brown rice - This is yet another popular choice of substrate for many first time cultivators. It does tend to get a little sticky and mushy during the process of sterilization but not as much as white rice would. Due to its availability, however, it is a good option to consider. I would heavily discourage using white rice, as it becomes too sticky and ends up one big, messy clump.

PSILOCYBIN MUSHROOMS

Popcorn - Surprisingly, a pretty good option if you do not mind the cost. It is almost always available in any grocery store, so you won't have problems finding it. The thing is, it can be a bit more expensive compared to others when buying in bulk. Another drawback is the size of the actual grain. They are quite large relative to other grains, which makes the inoculation period take a bit longer. The mycelium does not only have to cover the grains but bridge the significantly larger gaps between them as well.

Barley - Another condenser to consider, however, many do not suggest using it at first. Unfortunately, some of us cannot get a hold of something else and have no choice. The reason barley might not be the best option is due to it being very mushy and wet, with the grains breaking apart easily.

Sorghum - More commonly used by commercial growers due to its availability in the market; however, you can use it as well. Sorghum is usually used in animal feed, so if you have a commercial producer near you or know someone in that line of work, it can be a great option.

Millet - The smallest grain on this list. Due to the size of each grain, it is normally mixed in with other grains to provide a wider area of inoculation in the substrate. It mixes well with any other grains, so should you be short on one or the other, mix in some millet!

WBS -Wild bird seed is quite common amongst first-time growers and hobbyist growers. This is due to the cheap price tag on large bags of it. Unfortunately, the seeds are very inconsistent and do not really hold moisture all that well. Another thing to consider is that not all species enjoy this option, so you might end up with either a small yield or no yield. However, if you have no other choice, just find a compatible species, and you are good to go.

Wood Chips and Sawdust

If you really want to grow a wood-loving species, you will obviously have a wood-based substrate. When going this route, there is usually the nonsterile option as well. This is due to the nature of the substrate itself, as well as the fact that it is usually used outside.

The main reason for certain species to take a liking towards wood is due to lignin. It is basically the organic polymers forming key structural materials within plants. Therefore, a wood rich in lignin will be best suited.

The process for inoculation and the eventual transfer of the mycelium is also quite different from other methods, but we will get to that later. Either way, you will still need to make sure about the type of wood chips you will be using.

Alder Wood chips - This is the most popular choice for someone looking to go the wood chip route. So far it has had the best results for most cultivators compared to other wood chips.

Pine - This is not the best option for magic mushroom cultivation, but it does work. The best option would be to mix in some grain with it, however.

Maple - Also a good option, but not as popular. In general, people mix their wood with grain to get the best results, so there is not much information about the use of just wood itself. This is due to the inoculation process, but if you are confident enough, anything is possible.

Sawdust - Many people think that sawdust is a good option for growing their mushrooms. While this is not completely wrong, it is not completely right either. Using just sawdust will yield poor results, as the amount of nutrients available is minimal. The best option would be using a form of grain and then mixing the sawdust with the inoculated substrate.

The TEKs

These are methods for growing magic mushrooms either in jars or small containers, known as cakes. The reason for the existence of different TEKs is simply specialized substrates. When we go through cultivation methods step by step, you will understand the difference between growing a cake in a jar and using grain spawn.

PF-TEK, for example, also uses brown rice. The biggest difference is that vermiculite is mixed with the sterilized rice. The base in this TEK is vermiculite, which is basically hydrated minerals for the mushrooms. Not only that, but the shape, form, composition, and surface of vermiculite makes the best mycelium growth medium.

Decide on a Fruiting Chamber Setup

So, you have your substrate ready; now you will have to decide on the exact setup you will use for a fruiting chamber. If you already have a setup in mind, then you can skip to the steps of each method. I would suggest, however, to at least go through the differences of each setup so you can be sure you have the optimal method chosen for your species and/or substrate.

Some setups might require a bit more work than others. You will simply have to decide on what setup will be the best fit for you. I will also give a brief explanation of the setup I use after a few tries. It seems to work for me, so might work for you as well.

Monotub/Storage Tote

Seen as one of the more popular setups for cultivation, the monotub provides the best overall experience to most who try it for the first time. This setup usually has one tub or storage container. It can be of varying sizes, from a small 2-liter container to a larger 80 liter; either way, it will all depend on the amount you are looking to grow.

The best substrate selection for this would be grain spawn. You are able to spread out the grain evenly throughout the tub in order to get maximum colonization.

Some opt for a few medium-sized containers as they are a bit more manageable than the larger ones. As a bonus, you will be able to cultivate more than one strain. You will have to look out for cross-contamination in that situation, however.

The containers will need some holes cut into the sides in order to facilitate fresh air exchange so that the substrate does not dry out. It is possible to set it up with no holes, but it is generally accepted as a better option to have the holes. The bottom part up to about halfway on the sides is usually covered with either black paint, tape, paper, or any form of coverage that will block out light.

Some online stores even sell the tubs premodified so that you do not have to go through the trouble. I will be going through the steps to modify it yourself, however.

The basic idea behind the monotub is simple. You get your grain spawn or TEK, spread it at the bottom of the tub, and mix it with a bulk substrate like manure, wood chips, or mulch. The lid will be closed, the substrate will be colonized, and eventually, they will grow. You will have to open it every now and then in order to spritz it with water to keep humidity optimal.

That is the basic rundown on using a monotub; the detailed steps will come later.

Shotgun Fruiting Chamber (SGFC)

This setup is quite similar to the monotub in a few ways, as it uses a single tub or tote as well. The difference comes in with the function it provides inside the tub, as well as how everything is physically set up.

The SGFC must be clear throughout, unlike the basic monotub that blocks out light. Similar to the basic tub, this one needs holes cut into the sides; however, it will need holes on the lid and bottom as well. The best method is to have small holes drilled in a grid formation. The tub will also have to be raised from the ground. You can do this by either fashioning legs for it to stand on or cables to suspend it from something.

Damp perlite is then placed right at the bottom, with no spores or substrate yet. The idea behind this is that a natural air flow coupled with humidity will create the perfect environment for the mushrooms to cultivate. The substrate with the inoculated grain will then be spread over the damp perlite.

Due to this system, it cannot sit flat on a surface as it will block the airflow from the bottom. Fresh air will flow in through the bottom, rising up through the damp perlite. This system will assist in evaporation, which will bring the humidity up. This system works so well because humid air rises. It goes up and out, dragging fresh air in right behind it.

It is the perfect system for circulating fresh air without compromising on humidity.

Greenhouse

This setup is a bit too expensive for first-time cultivators, and sometimes even for experienced cultivators. The idea behind it is to create the perfect all-around environment for the mushrooms to grow.

I used a combination of the greenhouse method and monotub for my first grow, simply because I already had some of the supplies needed.

What many people seem to think when the word greenhouse comes up is a large shed-like construction. In fact, you are able to make a greenhouse in your own cupboard if you really want to. The term greenhouse is simply there to describe an enclosed space where the regulation of humidity and airflow are optimal for whichever species is being grown.

PSILOCYBIN MUSHROOMS

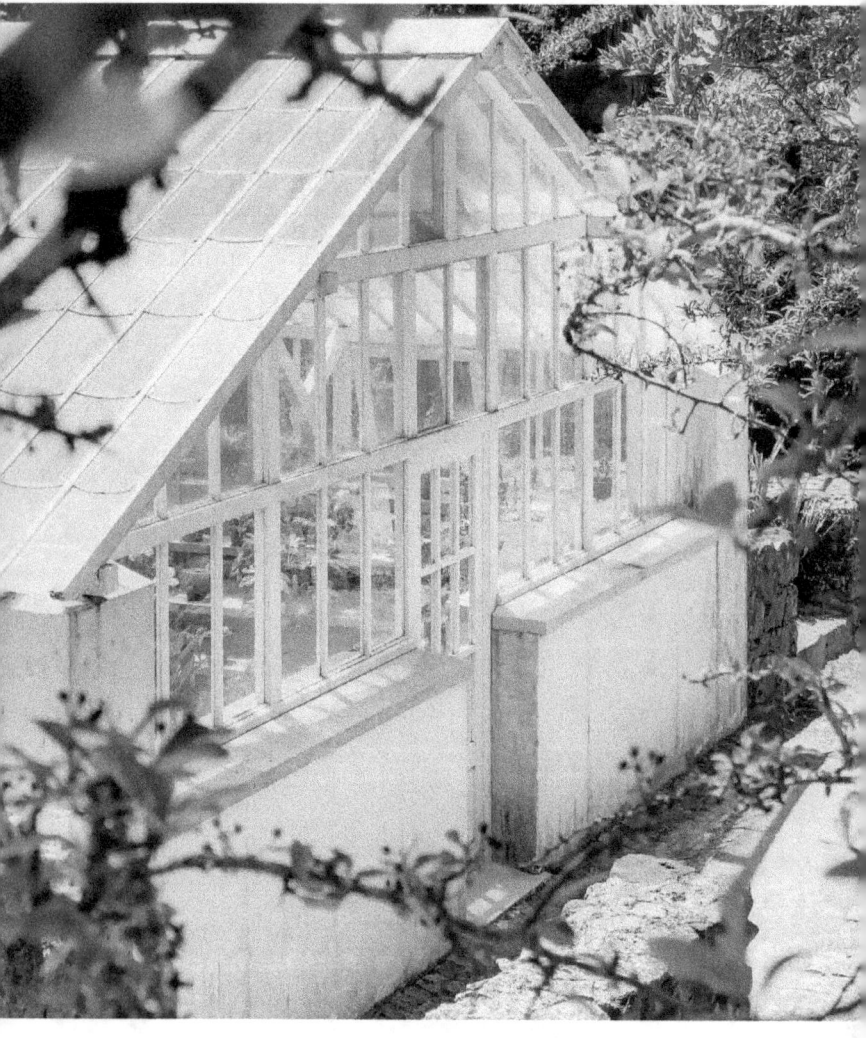

This is by far the most expensive setup, as the equipment needed can vary quite a lot depending on your build. Here is a list of popular equipment used:

- humidifiers (ultrasonic or filter type)
- piping and air ducting
- frames and materials depending on the structure shape and size
- fans
- water pumps
- temperature controllers
- light bulbs
- electrical wiring

These are a few basic equipment types that might be needed to build a proper greenhouse setup. While it might be costly, if you are looking to grow at a constant pace, it will be worth the investment.

This type of setup can be used in combination with any other; it will all depend on your experience and willingness.

Poor Man's Method

Let's face it, not all of us have the finances to buy something for a new setup, the last of which most likely went into getting the spores. There are basic setup options for you! While they are not always guaranteed to work, the basic principle is still there.

The Bag - This setup is quite literally just a plastic bag. Many first timers choose this method, especially when they have not done a lot of research. The inoculated grain spawn is thrown into a bag and then mixed with some soil. After it is mixed properly, the bag is simply placed somewhere in a cupboard. You open it every now and then to spritz it with water, and that is about it. In the end, it can work (50/50), so long as everything was sterilized.

The Jar/Can - Similar to the bag, it is just a small container that you can, essentially, throw all the necessary ingredients into and hope for the best. You can use recycled glass jars or tin cans for this setup.

Bottles - You can use plastic bottles cut in half to try and cultivate your mushrooms as well. It is basically the same as the monotub setup, just smaller. The yield will obviously be less, but it will get the job done.

Look, essentially you just need something to contain the inoculated substrate and mix it with a bulk substrate. Give the mushrooms the right amount of nutrients, water, and environment, then they will grow. A "poor man" can figure anything out.

Personal Setup

Here I will give you a quick rundown of my personal setup; you can decide if it will work for you or not. It will also give you an idea of just how creative you can be with your own setup if you understand the principles of the cultivation process.

I was able to cordon off a part of my garage for this setup. Basically, I used plastic sheeting, taped at the bottom to the floor and at the top to the ceiling. After a while, I was able to change it and seal it properly, as the tape kept coming off. The space was big enough for me to do all the inoculation work and have three medium-sized monotubs inside. The idea behind the space is to have a small secluded and sterile environment that you can keep clean easily. I added fans to the plastic to regulate airflow through filters. The monotubs were set up with three holes on each of the longer sides and two on each of the shorter sides.

I have a frame around the tubs so that I can place larger tubs upside down over the smaller FCs instead of a lid. The larger tubs had holes in a grid formation, similar to an SGFC.

Any setup can become expensive, the more equipment you add to it; luckily, I had the leftover plastic sheeting from a project my father worked on.

While the setup is not overly complicated, it provides a good all-around environment without actually constructing a complete greenhouse. So if you have space, you can always try your own setup.

A Step-by-Step Guide

Finally, we are here! This is where the magic happens, so to speak. I will be going over all of the methods listed above in a step-by-step formation. Some require more effort whereas others require minimal effort. It will all depend on the method you have chosen.

If you are confident in your own experiences and knowledge, you can always customize the steps to form your own method.

Without further ado, let's get started!

Monotub and Grain Spawn Method

We will be breaking up this method of cultivation into four main phases.

- **Phase 1** - Preparation of your setup
- **Phase 2** - Inoculation of your substrate
- **Phase 3** - The transfer
- **Phase 4** - Growth and care

Necessities:

Before we start with phase 1, however, let's go over everything you will need for this method. While it will depend on your substrate, I will be going over most of them, so not to worry.

1. **Latex gloves** - This is purely for sanitation and sterilization purposes. The whole process needs to

be kept as clean and sterile as possible; otherwise, contamination might occur. More than one pair is preferred.

2. **Paper towels** - You will be doing a lot of wiping down, so best to have enough ready

3. **A face mask** - The same as with the gloves but also for your own protection. You don't want to inhale any spores later during the process.

4. **Hairnet** - If you have a lot of hair, it would be best to wear a hairnet; you don't want your hair falling into anything, contaminating it.

5. **Rubbing alcohol (isopropyl alcohol)** - This will be used for cleaning almost everything, so it will be best to have enough ready for use.

6. **Mushroom spores** - The spores that you have will obviously depend on the species you have chosen. If you were able to get spore syringes, then great! They are the easiest to use, making inoculation a swift process. If you have spore prints, however, you will have to rehydrate them first which is a difficult process. The process will be described in the harvesting chapter. For now, a syringe will be what you need.

7. **Hypodermic needles** - Some syringes come with the needle, others do not. You will have to make sure if you have a needle; otherwise, you will have to go get one that fits your syringe. You cannot use

the syringe without one in this method; the risk of contamination is too high.

8. **A lighter (fire)** - This will be used to sterilize the needle without melting it. Matches will work as well, just not as great.

9. **Disinfectant spray** - This can be in any form; you can even make your own. Most people either buy some Lysol or make some with sterile water and isopropyl alcohol, which they just put in a spray bottle (you will need a lot).

10. **Water** - Obviously, you will need some water. A bottle you can use to spritz your mushrooms and substrate is the best option. Too much water is bad and too little water is bad. It cannot be tap water, as there are too many contaminants—use bottled water. If you cannot help but use tap water, boil it first.

11. **Monotub/storage tote** - this will be the fruiting chamber and is the biggest part of the whole setup. You can get a small- to medium-sized one depending on how much substrate you will have.

12. **Drill or knife** - This will be used to modify your tub with holes on the sides.

13. **A good spot** - Be sure to pick out a spot where all this will go down. You want a space that is small enough to manage and keep clean easily. You will need plenty of indirect sunlight as well.

14. **Temperature and humidity gauge** - While this is not a necessity, it will depend on the species you have selected. Most species will grow in a varied range of temperatures and humidity levels, while others are a lot more sensitive. My advice is to at least have a thermometer to gauge the temperature of the selected spot. The humidity you will always be able to regulate more easily with your spritzing bottle. Of course, having both does make it easier.

15. **Substrate and bulk substrate** - For this method, we will be using grain spawn. You will be able to get sterile and sealed grain packs from the same place you got your syringe, most likely. If not, however, simply pick a type of grain to use, and we will go over the sterilization process together. The bulk substrate can be any form of mulch, compost, coco coir, or perlite. You can buy sterilized and sealed bags of these as well from mushroom cultivation shops online or in your area.

16. **A jar and injection port** - This will only be necessary if you were unable to find already sterilized and sealed grain. Any glass jar with a sealable lid will do. Injection port you will be able to buy at a pharmacy or any store with lab and medical equipment. It is easier to find online, however.

17. **Paint and tape**- While the paint is not completely necessary, it does make harvesting later on easier. It is just to black out the bottom half of the fruiting

chamber, so spray paint is a popular option. You can use the tape for that as well. You will need the tape for other reasons though, so be sure to have enough. Duct tape works best.

18. **Poly-fill** - If you do not know what poly-fill is, it is basically synthetic cotton. It's that soft, cloudy-looking white stuff inside pillows, beds, and teddy bears. Many shops sell packs of it so no need to kill your teddy for it.

19. **Cardboard box** - While you do not necessarily need a box, any dark container will do. It is for placing your pack/jar of grain in after inoculation. So, a cupboard will be fine as well. Just be sure whatever it is, it is big enough. You do not want to run around looking for storage space after inoculation has been completed.

Phase 1: Preparation

Let's get started!

Step One A - FC modification

While many prefer modifying their fruiting chamber (FC) later on, I suggest you get it done first thing. Why not just do it and be done with it, right? Then all of the heavy work is finished.

So, what you want to do is get the drill and/or knife to make a total of 6–10 holes on the sides of your FC—either two or three holes on each of the longer sides, and one or two on each of the smaller sides. The number of holes will depend on the size of your FC: a bigger container means more holes. They can be between 2–4 inches across but not too big as you will have to close them up with poly-fill later on. Space them evenly from each other, more to the top half of the FC.

If you have paint, you can black out the bottom half of your container as well. The idea behind this is that the mushrooms will only grow out the top. Otherwise, if sunlight reaches through the bottom part of the container, it might start growing inside. That can make harvesting quite difficult later on.

Keep in mind the amount of substrate you will be using. Black out from the bottom upward. Either a fourth or third of the container, all depending on how much it will be filled.

Step One B - The jar

While you are waiting for the paint to dry, you might as well modify the jar for your grain (if you did not get a sterile and sealed pack). You will have to make a hole in the lid where you can then insert the injection port. It is fairly easy; just make sure not to make the hole too big. Using a drill for this usually works the best but not everyone has a drill. If you only have a knife, make sure the hole is smoothed out so it doesn't damage the injection port. You can always go to a hardware store and ask them to drill the holes for you; many stores provide such basic services for a small fee.

Step Two - Sterilization

Get all of your items ready and into the spot you decided to use. Many people decide on a bathroom, but that only works if you have more than one bathroom. If you perhaps have a shower and bathtub separate, you can use the tub as your space. Otherwise, find a corner in the smallest room you have available. So long as there is sunlight in the room itself, it will work.

It is at this point you will start sterilizing everything. Don your face mask, hair net, and gloves. You can start by cleaning all work surfaces with spray or rubbing alcohol and paper towels. All of the containers and sealed packs you have—items like the syringe, gauges, everything!

One of the most important things in all of the methods is keeping everything as clean and sterile as possible. Spray some disinfectant in the air regularly as well while you are cleaning.

Throw the gloves away when you are done with the cleaning process.

Step Three - If you have presterilized packs of grain and substrate, you can skip to Phase 2.

In order to sterilize your grain, you will have to leave it either in a steamer or pressure cooker for a few hours, and take it out just before the grain bursts open. This process can sometimes be a bit messy, depending on the grain used.

When it comes to the bulk substrate, however, many people just use a slow cooker for a few hours. If you have sealable containers to place the bulk substrate in, you can use them after they have been sterilized, of course. If not, you can just complete the process right before you move your inoculated grain over to the FC.

In the end, the idea is to make sure there is no bacteria or other spores caught in between your cultivation process.

You will have to sterilize your jar for the grain as well. Some people simply give it a proper wash and then rub it down with isopropyl alcohol. Others prefer to place the jar in a steamer or pressure cooker with the grain inside, or individually. It is up to you; just make sure it is cleaned right before putting the sterile grain inside. Close the lid right after filling it up with your sterilized grain. You can even seal it up with some tape if you want to.

I highly suggest getting sterilized packs of both your grain and bulk substrate for first-time cultivation. It makes the process much easier and reduces the chances of contamination by a large margin. As you build your experience, you can start experimenting with your own substrate sterilization and combinations.

Phase 2: Inoculation

Here comes the good stuff!

Step One - Sterilization and inoculation

PSILOCYBIN MUSHROOMS

So, now you have either your sealed pack of presterilized grain or your jar of self-sterilized grain. Both of them should have a self-healing injection port. When you enter your sterilized workspace, be sure to have some gloves on and spray some disinfectant on them.

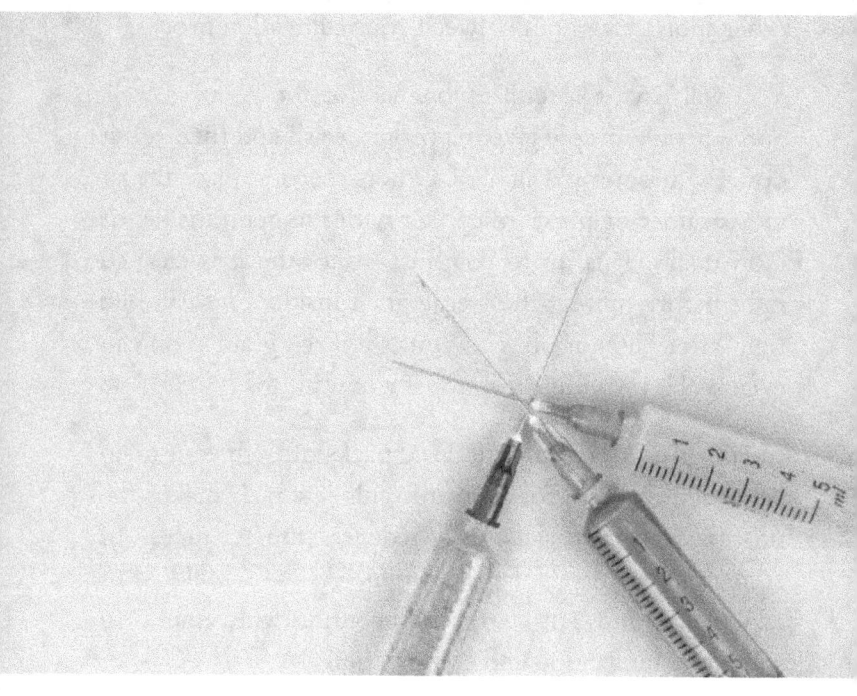

PSILOCYBIN MUSHROOMS

Wipe down the pack/jar of grain, specifically on the injection port. Take your syringe and wipe it down as well. Take your lighter and heat up the needle part of your syringe. Keep it there until the needle is red hot. While most of them do come presterilized, it's just in case. Once it is heated up, do not put the syringe down; keep it in your hand and wait for it to cool down. Once it has cooled down, you can shake it a bit to distribute the spores inside evenly.

Insert the needle into the injection port of your pack/jar at an angle. Inject about 1 cc into it and pull it out; you can put it back in at a different angle and inject another cc in. You can repeat this until the syringe is finished, or you can just inject everything in one go. Using different angles is just to make sure that the spores are spread evenly throughout the pack/jar.

If you have more than one pack/jar, just make sure to distribute the spores evenly between them.

Step Two - Patience

At this point, all you will have to do is simply wait. After inoculation of your grain, you will have to place the pack/jar into your box, container, or cupboard. Be sure it is dark and relatively warm, around 70 to 80 degrees should be fine. Do not be tempted to open the container to look at your pack/jar. The dark is needed for the mycelium to form.

After about five days, you are allowed to take a peek inside. If you see fuzzy white stuff starting to form inside your pack/jar, gently place it back into the dark container and close it up.

You may now do a small and contained victory dance!

The fuzzy stuff is mycelium; seeing it form is a good sign, but you will have to wait a bit longer before moving over to the next phase. The whole pack/jar needs to be colonized. You will have to be a bit more patient for about 10 to 15 days. It all depends on the species and grain. A bigger-sized grain will take longer to colonize.

Phase 3: The Transfer

This is where most of the work is done!

Step One - Finishing the fruiting chamber (FC)

On the last day or so of your grain being colonized, you will have to finish the modifications of your FC. You can even finish it up right before taking out the grain spawn. I just don't like finishing it up way before the time, as that leaves the poly-fill out in the open to contaminate.

So, what you will be doing is, again, sterilizing the FC with some spray and paper towels. All of this needs to be done while wearing gloves and the mask! Get the poly-fill and wipe down the bag. Open it and take out clumps of it. If you have the kind that is flattened out and rolled up, you will need some scissors to cut it into squares. Remember to wipe down the scissors as well!

If you have the clumps, take enough of it to fill up the holes you made; each hole needs to be filled. This will basically act as an air filter for the holes of the FC. If you have the flat type, simply cut out some squares big enough to cover the holes. Use the tape to secure both the clumps and/or squares to the FC. You do not want them falling out or into the FC.

At this point, you can give the FC a wipe down if you want, or leave it for just before you transfer the grain spawn. What you have to do, however, is spray the clumps/squares of poly-fill with some disinfectant.

Step Two - Transferring the grain spawn

This is where everything gets real. You will have to bring your pack/jar of colonized grain into your workspace. Rub down the pack/jar again, as well as the inside of the FC. While some people prefer to put the grain first, I like to add a bit of the bulk substrate into the FC first. You do not have to put in a lot—just enough to cover the bottom surface of the FC.

If you have a sealed pack of the bulk substrate, give it a quick rubdown again, as well as the knife you use to cut it open. Pour some into the FC and spread it evenly across the surface. Place the bag on the side where you can reach it easily.

If you have a pack of grain spawn, you can try to break it apart through the sealed pack. You will notice it is quite stiff, almost like the grains are glued together. Breaking them apart will not damage the mycelium, but it will make it easier to spread out evenly in the FC. Do this before cutting a hole into the pack.

If you have a jar, you will obviously not be able to break it apart like that. You might have some difficulty getting it out of the jar as well. It will depend on the grain used, as some will come apart easier than others. If you do struggle, you can use the sterilized knife to try and break apart the grains to take them out.

Now you can start taking bits and pieces of the clumped grains and spreading them evenly over the first layer of substrate in the FC. Do not use all of it at once—the objective is to create an even multilayered cake. Once the first layer is done, add some of the bulk substrate again. You can start spritzing some water over it as well; this will add more moisture to the substrate, not too much though. The last thing you want is one big gooey mess.

Add the next layer of grain spawn, spread evenly over the second layer of the substrate. Keep in mind that these layers of substrate are not very thick, just enough to cover the grain spawn. Do this until all the grain spawn is used. All in all, the whole cake should not be thicker than 4 inches. The ideal thickness is between 2 and 3 inches.

After this whole process is done, you can give it a last few spritzes of water. Remember, the mycelium has been going at your grain in an airtight pack/jar. It will need something to drink. A good way to measure the moisture is to grab a handful of the substrate and squeeze it. While the water should not be pouring out, you should be able to see at least a drop or two come out.

You can now close the lid—be sure to spray and wipe down the lid before closing, however. After closing the lid, do not open it again. You can look through the sides or the top, but opening the lid will just risk contamination.

Be sure the level of light in the room is kept at a minimum for at least a week after the transfer.

Step Three - Casing

In about a week or two, you will notice a layer of mycelium growing over the top of your substrate, which means all is going well. Do not open it up yet, though.

Keep an eye out for small pins starting to form. This should happen right around the two-week mark, and depending on the species, it can happen sooner or later. Now you may open your lid; the risk for contamination is mostly over. Do not take that as a sign to sneeze into the container or take it outside, however. You still have to try and be as clean as possible, but the wipe downs will not be necessary anymore.

You can now start casing your substrate with some materials, depending on the species of mushroom you chose. If you have a wood-loving species, wood chips will be best. Other species might enjoy some sterilized compost, bark, some coco cair, perlite or mulch. This step is not necessary, but it can help increase the size of your yield.

Depending on what materials you have access to and the species of mushroom you chose, you can ignore the casing part.

You can cover the layer of mycelium with about half an inch of your chosen materials. Spritz some water over it when you are done; be sure it is nice and moist. You can also decide not to add anything, but you will still need to spritz some water over the existing substrate and mycelium.

Step Four - Position of the FC

Whether you cased your mycelium in other materials or not, you will have to double-check on the placement of your FC from this point on. You need to be sure there is enough sunlight inside the room itself. No direct sunlight should be shining into the FC at all, however.

Imagine that shady little corner that almost everyone has in their room. The sun comes in through your window, but it will always miss the corner; it never gets exposed to direct sunlight. That is the type of spot you have to look for.

The mushrooms will be growing toward the sunlight, which is why they go up. The blacking out of the bottom part of your FC will make sure they grow the way nature intended.

Phase 4 - Growth and Care

Where everything starts to pay off!

So, at this stage of the process, you can almost be certain that you will have some nicely growing magic mushrooms in just a few days. You will have to keep the humidity up in your FC for the duration of the fruiting period.

You can do this by misting the chamber with water between two and four times a day. Some people close their lids up again completely every time, while others keep them open about halfway. This will all depend on the amount of airflow you have in the area you chose.

If there is minimal airflow, like in most bathrooms, I would suggest keeping the door and a window open. You can even opt for a standing fan or extractor fan in the room. You will have to keep the lid open just a little bit—not too much, however; you do not want to dry out your new babies.

If you feel the airflow is regulated enough throughout the area you have decided to place your FC, then you can keep the lid closed. The holes you made will ensure enough fresh air for the mushrooms to grow. You can swap out some of the poly-fill for new clumps and/or squares every few days as well, but it is not necessary.

So long the humidity is kept between 50%–100%, it should be ok. It is preferred, however, to keep the humidity level around 80%–90%. That is the perfect ratio for most species of psilocybe mushrooms.

You will have to keep an eye on the temperature as well during this period. The optimal temperature for mushrooms to grow, depending on species, can range from 60 to 85 degrees. Most people argue, however, that the best temperature is about 70 degrees.

After about five days, depending on the species, you should see a few mushrooms starting to grow from the substrate. You will still have to mist them for a few days, but harvesting them is right around the corner!

We will discuss the harvesting process in the next chapter; for now, let's take a look at another method of cultivation.

Shotgun Fruiting Chamber(SGFC) and Cake Method

We will be breaking up this method of cultivation into four main phases, the same as with the monotub setup. While the phases might look the same, they differ from each other when it comes to your setup and transfer.

- **Phase 1** - Preparation of your setup

- **Phase 2** - Inoculation of your jars

- **Phase 3** - Birthing and soaking

- **Phase 4** - Growth and maintenance

Necessities

Before we start, let's take a look at everything you will need for the SGFC method.

1. **Latex gloves, hairnet, face mask** - Exactly as with the previous setup, and most setups for that

matter. The whole process needs to be kept as clean and sterile as possible, otherwise. You have to try your best to avoid contamination, especially with the SGFC method.

2. **Paper towels** - As with the previous method, you will be doing a lot of wiping down, so best to have enough on hand.

3. **Rubbing alcohol (isopropyl alcohol)** - It is best to have quite a lot, especially if you make your own disinfectant spray.

4. **Mushroom spores** - You cannot do much without these. The spores that you have will obviously depend on the species you have chosen. I would suggest getting a syringe. They are the easiest to use, making inoculation a swift process.

5. **Hypodermic needles** - You cannot use the syringe without the needle in this method, the risk of contamination is too high. Make sure to have one ready.

6. **A lighter (fire)** - This will be used to sterilize the needle without melting it.

7. **Disinfectant spray** - While most people just buy some Lysol, you can make some with sterile water and isopropyl alcohol.

8. **Water** - Be sure to use bottled water. If you can only get tap water, boil it. Also, be sure to have a misting bottle as well.

9. **Monotub/storage tote** - This will be the main part of the fruiting chamber. The size will depend on your choice; just be sure it is manageable.

10. **Drill** - For the SGFC method, it is best to have a drill for modifications. The best-sized drill bit is about a quarter inch. While a knife will work, the number of holes you need to make is significantly more than with a normal monotub setup. You will be sitting around all day carving holes with a knife, but if it's all you have, then you can still do it.

11. **Marker/pencil** - While not necessary, it will make mapping out your grid on the monotub later on much easier. Anything that you can use to make a dot on the plastic tub will do.

12. **Tray** - You will need a tray that is of a bigger size compared to your monotub. While you don't have to worry about massive amounts of water leaking out, it is better to be prepared for everything.

13. **Frame** - You will need to build or find a frame for your SGFC to stand on. If you cannot build or find anything, try to get some books or bricks to place underneath the corners of the SGFC. The best and cheapest option to build a permanent frame, however, is using PVC conduit/piping. You will

need enough for the length and width of your SGFC. You will also need fittings for the corners (to connect them together); three-way fittings work best. You can find all of this at a local hardware store.

14. **Saw/cutting tool** - You will need something to cut the PVC conduit to the correct sizes. This can either be a type of saw or a power tool.

15. **A good spot** - As with the previous method, pick a good spot with no direct sunlight.

16. **Temperature and humidity gauge** - These two make the regulation of your SGFC much easier, but they are not necessary.

17. **Substrate** - For this method, we will be using a cake TEK. You are able to buy containers with a sterilized grain inside from most online mushroom cultivation shops. These containers can be either plastic or glass. The grain is usually a mixture of brown rice and brown rice flour. Most grains will do, however. Try to get a few small ones, as this method needs more than one cake. We will discuss a sterilization process if you could not find any online or in your area.

18. **Jars and injection ports** - This will only be necessary if you were unable to find already sterilized and sealed grain, or perhaps only one large one. Any glass jars with a sealable lid will do,

wide mouthed is a must. Try to get some on the smaller side (about 4–6 inches long and 3 inches wide), as you will be placing a few of them into the SGFC together. Injection ports can be found at any store online or in your area selling lab and medical equipment.

19. **Extra containers** - You will need a few extra containers big enough to contain the cakes that come out of the jars. They need to be watertight. Plastic bags will work as well as long as there are no holes in them.

20. **Perlite** - For the SGFC method to work, you will need some perlite. However, you will not need any other bulk substrate.

21. **Cardboard box** - While you do not necessarily need a box, any dark container will do. It is for containing your inoculated jar in a dark space. Just be sure whatever it is, it is big enough.

Phase 1: Preparation

Let's get started!

Step One A- Making the SGFC

When making the SGFC, there are a few things that you need to keep in mind. The whole idea behind going through all the effort in the first place is to make an FC that has natural air currents. In turn, the air currents will create high relative humidity and a constant flow of fresh air. This is known as fresh air exchange (FAE).

This whole system is designed to simulate the ideal environment for your mushrooms, so you have to be precise. You can start with either the lid or the tub itself; just keep in mind you will be doing all six sides, which means bottom and top as well.

Take your marker and start mapping out a grid of dots on the side you will be starting with. I usually suggest the lid, as you can always replace the lid easier than the tub if you make a mistake the first time around. Each hole should be around a quarter inch in diameter, spaced about two inches apart from each other. That means if you make a hole right in the middle of the lid, another should be two inches above it, another below it, another to the left, and another to the right.

When the lid is finished, you can start with all the other sides of your tub, including the bottom. Remember to keep the holes spaced evenly apart; otherwise, the FAE will not work.

Step One B - Your jars

After all the holes are finished, you can move on to the lids of your jars. This is only if you were unable to get some presterilized jars with a grain.

Simply drill holes into the center of all the lids for your jars. Be sure the holes are big enough for the injection ports to fit snugly. Going too big means they won't seal properly.

When all the drilling work is complete, you can put the drill away, clean up the shavings left on the floor, and move onto the next step.

Step One C - The frame

In this step, you will be making the frame for your SGFC to stand on. This is a vital step in the SGFC process; without it, the whole system will fall apart.

You do not necessarily have to BUILD a frame for the SGFC; you can just let it stand on a few bricks or books. Building a frame for it, however, will result in a more stable setup so that it does not accidentally fall over when bumped or moved.

PVC conduit is the best option, as it provides a stable enough frame, and is not difficult to work with. It is fairly cheap as well, compared to other materials. Start by measuring the bottom of your SGFC, the width, and the length. You will have to take into consideration the added length to the conduit when attaching the fittings.

The fittings should be three-way-fittings. This will allow you to connect the PVC pieces together in a rectangle formation, with the third side of each fitting pointing downward, functioning as a foot for the frame to stand on.

The frame should be about an inch smaller than the SGFC, depending on the overall size of the SGFC. For example, if the width of your SGFC is 10 inches and the length is 20 inches, the frame, with fittings, will have to measure in at about 9 inches wide and 19 inches long.

When finished, the SGFC should be able to sit on the frame in a stable position, with around 2–4 inches of space from the floor or surface you place it on. If the fittings alone are not enough to raise it to such a height, you can always just add some PVC conduit to increase the height.

If you feel like the SGFC is not stable enough on the frame, you can secure it to the frame. You can use some glue to stick the frame to the SGFC permanently if you want. Another option is to drill a few holes into the frame. You can then feed some zip-ties through the holes of the frame and SGFC to secure it that way. You can always cut the zip-ties later on if you want to remove the frame.

Once everything is finished, you can move the SGFC and frame to your selected cultivation spot.

Step Two - Sterilization

Get everything ready and into the room or spot where you decided to set up your SGFC. Be sure there is a flat surface somewhere to place your tray; the SGFC and frame will have to stand on that tray.

It is at this point you will start sterilizing everything the same as with the previous method. Don your face mask, hair net, and gloves. You can start by cleaning all work surfaces with spray or rubbing alcohol and paper towels—

all of the containers and sealed packs you have, items like the syringe, gauges, everything! This includes the tray!

One of the most important things in all of the methods is keeping everything as clean and sterile as possible. This is even more applicable to the SGFC, as there will be no poly-fill to filter the holes.

Throw the gloves away when you are done with the cleaning process, and remember to spray some disinfectant into the air every now and then.

Step Three - If you have presterilized jars and grain for your cake, you can skip to Phase 2.

You will have to sterilize your grain if you were unable to get some presterilized grain. This can be done with a pressure cooker or steamer, same as with the previous method.

You will also have to sterilize your jars for the grain. You can simply give them a proper wash and then rub them down with isopropyl alcohol. If you have a steamer or pressure cooker, you can place them in there as well. This method is quite outdated, however, but it still works.

Remember to sterilize the jars right before your grain is finished sterilizing; then you can move everything into the jars and seal them up nice and tight.

I highly suggest getting presterilized jars with a grain. It just makes the process much easier and reduces the chances of contamination. This is especially true for first-time cultivators.

Phase 2: Inoculation of your jars

Very similar to the previous method

Step One - Sterilization and inoculation

So, now you have a few jars of self-sterilized or presterilized grain, great! They should all have injection ports by now.

Wipe down the jars with disinfectant, focusing on the injection ports. Be sure to have your mask and gloves on at this point. Take your syringe and wipe it down as well. Use your lighter or another flame source to heat up the needle part of your syringe. It has to be red hot; otherwise, there is no point. Most of them do come presterilized, but you can never be too careful. Once it is heated up, do not put the syringe down; keep it in your hand and wait for it to cool. Once it has cooled down, you can shake it a bit to distribute the spores inside evenly.

Start with one jar at a time, and press the needle into the injection port of your jar. Inject about 1 cc into it and pull it out. This will depend on how many syringes and jars you have; try to divide the amount equally between the jars. If you have more than one syringe, start with just one, sterilize the needle, and use it until it is finished. Throw it to the side, sterilize the next needle, wipe down the injection ports of the jars next in line while it's cooling in your hand, and continue. You can use different angles of injection, similar to the first method.

Try to move as quickly as possible between the jars to get them all ready.

Step Two - Waiting

After the initial inoculation of your jars, you will have to place them into your box, container, or cupboard. Be sure it is dark and relatively warm, around 70 to 80 degrees. Do not open the container to look at the progress of your jars. The dark is needed for the mycelium to form.

After about five days, you are allowed to take a peek inside. If you see the mycelium start to form inside your jars, then great! If you see the mycelium only forming in some of the jars, just leave them be for now.

Each jar needs to be colonized. After about another five to 15 days they should all be colonized. If for some reason some jars are colonized and others not, you will have to assume the ones that have no growth are botched and throw them out.

If you do see some growth in a few of them (say halfway colonized), you can decide to leave them for now. You can then take out the fully colonized ones. Keep in mind, if you put them all in the SGFC together, growth will be more even throughout.

If you leave some of the jars, you will have to place the cakes in the SGFC later on, which will hinder the cakes already inside. It will also increase the risk of contamination. The growth of the mushrooms will be uneven as well.

Phase 3: Birthing and Soaking

There are a few differences in the steps from the previous method.

Step One - Birth and soak

Oaky, so you have your fully colonized jars. Now it's time to "birth" them.

Keep in mind, the mycelium is now almost dried out as it's been colonizing in an airtight container. Due to the fact that we will not be placing any extra bulk substrate over the grain spawn, we will have to soak the cakes first.

This is where your extra watertight containers or plastic bags come in, so keep them right next to you. You will also need enough bottled or sterile water to soak all of them. You will also need a flat surface or tray in front of you. You can use the tray set out for the SGFC; just make sure you spray and wipe it down properly.

First, you can start with putting on new gloves and your mask. Start with only one jar at a time, and spray and wipe down the jar. Open the lid slowly and place it on the side away from the lid. Turn the jar around over the tray. If you are lucky, the cake will come out easily, if not… you will have to bang it on the tray a bit. You can tap it on the back with your hand as well. The cakes should be fairly solid, so they won't just fall apart.

Once you finally get the cake out, move it over to the plastic bag or container (be sure the bag/container was wiped down inside and out beforehand). Fill the container/bag with the sterile water, as full as possible. The cake will most likely float, so if you can fill it up completely and seal it, that would be best. Using a bag for this can be difficult, but just make sure to force out as much air as you possibly can.

Do this for each and every cake. While some do not mind placing the cakes in the same container to soak, I prefer to use separate ones. You never know what contaminants might be in one or the other.

Once you are finished with all of your cakes, you will have to make room in your refrigerator. Place them in there to soak between 12–24 hours. You can basically just leave them overnight, and move on to the next step in the morning.

Step Two - Prepare the SGFC

You will want to complete this step right before taking your cakes out of the fridge. Get the perlite and a big container you can soak it in. A few small containers can work as well.

While some people prefer to put the perlite in a slow cooker first, it doesn't really do much. What you can do instead is mix some isopropyl alcohol or hydrogen peroxide with sterile water; the ratio should be around 10 parts water and 1 part of the other. Soak the perlite in this mixture for a few minutes; this will get rid of any dust from the perlite as well as other bacteria and spores. You can use your hands (while wearing gloves) to slosh the perlite around in the water. After washing the dust off, you can either drain the water in order to add new water or leave it as is to soak.

Remember, the main reason for the perlite being there is to maintain humidity.

While the perlite is soaking, you can go to spray and wipe your SGFC and tray. Put the tray on a flat surface with the SGFC on top of it.

The order should be as follows: floor/flat surface - tray - frame/stand - SGFC.

When done, you can drain the water from your perlite and start spreading it evenly inside your SGFC. Now, there might be some perlite falling out the bottom of your SGFC; don't worry about that, the tray is there for a reason.

Fill up the SGFC until there is a layer of perlite about 4 inches thick. You can take the tray out once you are finished as it most likely has some perlite on it. You can throw it into the SGFC, or you can throw it out, your choice. Remember to put the tray back, however.

Step Three -Transferring the cakes

Once your SGFC is set up properly and the perlite is even, you can transfer your cakes. Take your containers out of the fridge and bring them into the room/area your SGFC is located. Give them all a quick spray and wipe down.

Remember your gloves and mask.

If you kept the lids for your jars, you can place them on the perlite, spaced evenly apart (remember to spray and wipe the lids first). You will be putting the cakes right on top of them, so make sure there is enough space between them for growth. If you did not keep the lids, it's okay. They make harvesting easier and less messy, as the cakes will not fuse with the perlite, but it is not a necessity.

Start with one cake at a time. Open up the container, take the cake out, and let some of the water drip off. While you have it in your hand, give it a quick sniff. If it smells normal, as in like a fresh mushroom type of smell, then all is well. You can place it gently on one of the lids or straight onto the perlite.

If it smells odd, foul, or sour, it means that the cake is most likely contaminated with harmful bacteria. It is highly recommended that you throw it out. You do not want to place it in the SGFC with the others. If you do not want to waste it either, you can try to grow it in a different container in a separate space. If the smell gets worse over a few days, throw it out, as it can be a major health risk.

Okay, once all the cakes are sitting comfortably in the SGFC, spritz/mist them with some sterile water and close the lid.

Step Four - Position of the SGFC

Always double check the placement of your SGFC. You need to be sure there is enough sunlight inside the room itself. No direct sunlight should be shining into the SGFC, however.

You can also use this time to check that the tray is in place properly and the SGFC is placed correctly on its frame. You do not want it to fall over when you are not there or accidentally bump it over.

Something else to consider is the airflow inside the room. Due to the design of the SGFC, it already facilitates a natural FAE, so you cannot put a fan in the room. That will dry out your cakes very quickly.

Phase 4 - Growth and Maintenance

Fairly similar to the first method—however, there are key differences to look out for.

If you have temperature and humidity gauges, you will want to check them regularly. The best temperature is 70–75 degrees, with the best humidity being 80%–90%.

If you notice some condensation on the inside of the SGFC, then the temperature inside the SGFC is higher than outside. This should not happen, and it means the

FAE is obstructed. You can try to open the lid a bit to help with this.

You will have to keep misting your cakes during the day, 3–6 times. Make sure they glisten every time, but do not soak them completely. What you can do when taking off the lid to mist the cakes is fan the SGFC. Simply take the lid and fan it a few times to clear all the air out of it. This will also help with preventing condensation.

You will most likely notice the pinning stage early on. With some species, this might even happen when first taking them out of their soaking containers. After a few days, they will start to grow. The time will depend on the species of mushroom, but usually, after five days you will start to see significant progress.

Harvesting will be discussed in the next chapter; for now, however, well done! You are almost there!

Outside Cultivation With Grain Spawn

The method for outside cultivation is not drastically different from that for the inside. The only difference will be that there is no fruiting chamber but rather an outdoor mushroom bed (OMB).

Here are the phases we will follow:

- **Phase 1** - Inoculation

- **Phase 2** - OMB preparation

- **Phase 3** - Growth and maintenance

Necessities

There are still a few things you will need even when cultivating outside; here is a list.

1. **Latex gloves** - You will still need to work in a clean environment when inoculating your grain, so it will be best to wear gloves

2. **Rubbing alcohol (isopropyl alcohol)** - For rubbing down the grain spawn packs and syringe

3. **Mushroom spores** - The best option is to get a few syringes with hypodermic needles.

4. **A lighter** - For sterilizing the needle.

5. **A good spot** - As with the previous methods, pick a good spot with no direct sunlight. This spot, however, will have to be outside where you can make an OMB.

6. **Substrate** - Getting a few presterilized grain packs is the best option. You will need a few, depending on the size of the OMB. For the bulk substrate, you will need some wood chips and something else to mix it with like mulch, soil, or compost. You will need some straw as well.

7. **Cardboard box** - You will need some cardboard when starting the OMB.

8. **Shovel** - For actually digging the OMB

Phase 1 - Inoculation

Basically the same as the other methods.

Step One - Sterilization and inoculation

Enter a small workspace you can clean and sterilize easily. Take your packs of presterilized grain and wipe them down as with previous methods, specifically on the injection port.

Take a syringe and wipe it down, and use the lighter to sterilize the needle. Inject your spores into the packs, depending on how many syringes and packs you have. You will have to distribute the spores evenly. As with the previous method, finish one syringe before moving on to the next. Wipe the injection ports before every injection.

Step Two - Waiting, again.

After inoculation of your packs, you can place them in a dark container or cupboard as with other methods. Keep the container closed for at least five days, after which you may check up on the packs.

If mycelium growth seems normal, then great! Leave them be for another few days until colonization is complete.

Phase 2 - OMB preparation

This is where the sweating starts!

Step One - Digging

When colonization is complete, you will have to start preparing your OMB. Head towards the spot you picked out for the OMB and start digging! The size will all depend on you; smaller is easier to manage, however.

It is better to wait for colonization to be almost finished before starting to dig. You never know what might happen with your OMB while waiting for colonization to complete.

Dig a square hole; about two feet deep should be fine. Layer the cardboard at the bottom and the sides—this will keep contamination to a minimum. It will also keep the weeds out. Digging the hole square simply makes layering the cardboard much easier, but any shape will do.

Be sure that this hole does not have direct sunlight shining on it! The placement should be somewhere with lots of shade, like under a tree, or roof.

Step Two - Layering

After the cardboard is laid out, you can start with a layer of wood chips and substrate.

After the first layer, you can take a pack of your grain spawn and start breaking it up. Open the pack and spread it evenly over the substrate. It will work very similarly to a normal monotub. Keep layering your grain spawn, wood chips, and substrate until it is all finished. You can spray a bit of sterile water mixed with isopropyl alcohol in between layers if you want to keep contamination to a minimum.

When you are finished, you can place a layer of straw over the OMB. Spray the layer of straw with sterile water. Make sure you soak it nicely, but not so much that puddles start forming.

You can also place some cardboard over the whole OMB for the first few days in order to keep the conditions optimal for the pins to start forming.

Phase 3 - Growth and maintenance

The growth period for mushrooms outside seems to vary quite a lot, so do not be surprised if you start seeing progress only a week or two later. The conditions are far more difficult to regulate compared to an inside setup. It will all depend on the species you decided on, but keep watering the top every day. Sterile water is preferred. If it rains, be sure the bed does not drown completely.

Once you start seeing the mushrooms breach the straw, you can let up on the watering and start to mist the mushrooms every day. It will almost be time to harvest!

Building a Greenhouse

If you want to build a greenhouse (GH) for your psilocybin mushrooms, I can help you with a basic setup! You can use the GH in combination with any of the above-mentioned methods.

A GH does not necessarily have to be outside, as you can make a hybrid version of it in your garage or another unused room.

PSILOCYBIN MUSHROOMS

Here are the phases to follow for a basic setup:

- **Phase 1** - Building the frames

- **Phase 2** - Adding the covering

- **Phase 3** - Installing other equipment

Necessities:

Here is a list of things you will require for a basic GH:

1. **Frame material** - You will have to decide on what type of material you want to build your frame with. For this build, we will be using PVC conduit, fittings, and steel rods.
2. **Covering** - You will have to decide on what type of coverage you will be using for the greenhouse. Plastic sheeting is the best option. You get a few options when it comes to the color and thickness of the sheeting, but clear is the best.
3. **Steel rods** - You will need some steel rod to place inside of the PVC frame. This will weigh it down a bit, as well as strengthen the integrity of the frame.
4. **Tools** - You will need tools to cut the PVC and steel rods; it can be either a saw or power tools. You will also need fasteners like zip-ties and some duct tape.
5. **Environment control equipment** - This will all depend on how much money you want to spend on the setup. If you want at least a basic level of autonomy, you will need a humidifier, ventilation fan, temperature gauge, and humidity gauge.

Phase 1 - Building the frames

The GH can be as large or as small as you want. I prefer one where I can at least turn around without bumping into something.

Step One - The frame

The most basic form I suggest is 6.5 feet for length and width. Seven feet should be fine for the height. It will literally just be a cube—easy to manage, assemble, and disassemble.

Start with measuring the PVC conduit and cutting them up. It should be about eight pieces measured at 6.5 feet and four pieces at 7 feet. Once that is finished, you can cut the steel rod as well. I suggest cutting the steel rods about a quarter inch shorter than the PVC.

- Start laying out the bottom part where you want the GH located.

- Place the PVC in a square formation.

- Insert steel rods into each conduit

- Attach each PVC to each other with three-way corner fittings.

- Start adding the pillar parts of each corner; leave the steel rods at first.

- Once all corners are up, you can insert the rods

- Build the top part of the frame on the ground in a similar fashion to the bottom and then attach it to the top after it is finished.

- The fittings should be reasonably secure, but you can tape them up if you want to.

Step Two - Shelving

You can make shelving for your tubs, depending on the number of tubs you want inside your GH. You can build them using the same method as building the frame. Be sure the shelving is able to fit inside the GH without obstructing movement.

A basic shelf can have three layers—the bottom, the middle, and the top. You can make the shelf about 5 feet high to make it manageable. You will have to make a grid on top and in the middle for the tubs to sit on; the bottom tubs can just sit on the floor.

Phase 2 - Adding the covering

The covering can be the more difficult part, but if you work in steps, you can finish quickly.

Step One - Top and bottom

Steps one and two will be fairly similar.

- Take your plastic covering/sheeting, roll it out to measure, and mark the length and width of the top and bottom. Add about an inch extra on each side.

- Cut out the squares and start out with one side at the top; tape it onto the frame with duct tape.

- You can poke a hole through the sheet to secure it with zip-ties if you prefer that.

- Pull the sheeting tight from the opposite side you taped it to.

- Now you can tape the side where you are pulling from. It does not have to be super tight; just enough tension to keep it straightened out.

- After the two sides are secure, you can tape the two remaining sides.

That is the top side done! You can now move on to the bottom side and follow the same steps. Just roll the frame over; it will be sturdy enough. The reason for using tape is to make deconstruction at a later time easier. It will also make replacing each sheet easier.

Step Two - The sides

You can now tape the other three sides. Leave one side open. Keep in mind that the height is longer than the other sides, so keep the correct side open!

Step Three - The door

- Roll out some sheeting and measure from the side to about an inch or two past the center of the frame.

- Make sure that it will be long enough to reach down from the top to the bottom. Make two of these pieces.

- You can now tape the one piece to the top, and then the second piece.

- Tape the sides to the frame as well but leave the bottom.

You will notice the two sheets cross each other in the center, which will be your "door." It does not seal completely, but it closes up after you pass through it.

Phase 3 - Installing other equipment

Now you have a basic greenhouse! You can start with the installation of your other equipment.

This phase will be up to you, as it will depend on the amount of equipment you have. What I suggest is installing a medium-sized extraction fan in one of the top corners of the GH at the back. Another medium-sized fan pulling in the fresh air will be perfect at the bottom corner. You can simply cut holes into the plastic and then secure the fans to the frame with tape or zip-ties.

If you have a humidifier, you can place it in the middle of the GH or in one of the corners. Placement will depend on how many shelves you will have.

I would also suggest running a power cable with a multi-plug into the GH. It just makes it easier to provide power to your equipment.

There you have it! A basic greenhouse setup where you can cultivate some psilocybin mushrooms! The plastic should also be cleaned when sterilizing the GH after every new grow.

You can customize this setup in any way you want. It is just a basic build for beginners looking to test out the waters.

It Is Not That Difficult

So, after you went through the methods of growing your own mushrooms, did you realize it? It really is not that difficult to grow your own. As long as you follow the steps you should be fine.

One thing to keep in mind throughout the whole process is to keep everything as clean as possible. Sterilize everything you can, as you never know what contaminants might be hiding where you are working. After the initial cultivation of your grain, the risk of contamination starts to go down. After you see pins start to form, you are basically there, and the risk lowers even more. Once you see actual growth, the risk is nearly completely gone.

PSILOCYBIN MUSHROOMS

It truly is worth it, however, to clean everything when you are busy. It might seem redundant, but there is nothing worse than finding out your mushrooms are contaminated after you went through all the effort of growing them in the first place.

CHAPTER 4

HARVESTING AND STORAGE

So, you have decided on a method to grow your mushrooms; who knows, you might have already started or even finished. Now you probably want to harvest those beautiful mushrooms!

I understand that you are most likely brimming with anticipation. Keep in mind that you have been patient all this time so no need to go crazy on the mushrooms now. You will have to work delicately; otherwise, you might damage the mushrooms. While that doesn't necessarily sound dangerous, it can be problematic for future cultivation.

The Harvesting Process

Okay, so there are a few things you need to know about the harvesting process before you can begin, so let's start with that. We will cover a range of precautions to follow when you start your process. These precautions aren't just for the safety of your mushrooms but for your personal safety as well.

Precautions

You will have to follow a few basic steps in order to prepare for harvesting, no matter the method of cultivation you used. Let's make a small list of things you will have to look out for when harvesting.

- You will have to be careful not to contaminate the substrate if you want to continue growing more mushrooms. We will discuss this in a bit more detail later on.

- You will have to pay close attention to the growth of your mushrooms. One night might be the difference between a good harvest and a room full of spores.

- Be careful of the spores once they are out; you do not want them all over the place, including your lungs. You can even release the spores yourself accidentally.

- Be prepared to store the mushrooms properly; otherwise, you might end up with rotten mushrooms later on. It's not like you will be able to eat them all at once anyway. We will discuss storage methods later on.

- If you want to make your own spore kits, you will have to be very attentive to the stages your mushrooms go through. We will discuss this in more detail later on as well, so not to worry.

Okay, those are the basics you will have to look out for while harvesting. Let's go over a list of things you will need when first starting to harvest.

Necessities

1. **Gloves and mask** - You will most likely have some left from your actual growing phase, and you will need them now as well. While you won't need them for sanitary reasons, you will need them for protection. It sounds a bit extreme, I know, but better safe than sorry, am I right?
2. **Tweezers** - When first starting out with the harvesting process, you might notice some discrepancies in the size of your mushrooms. While some might be quite large, others will be relatively small when compared to the others. It won't be that they need to grow some more, as they will most likely be ready to release their spores soon. That means you won't be able to wait much longer before harvesting them as well. So, you will need some tweezers.
3. **Scissors** - These will come in handy, trust me.
4. **Containers** - After harvesting your mushrooms, you will need something to put them in. You don't

want them lying around or falling on the floor—you're going to eat them after all. A bag or container will work for the initial harvesting phase; no lid is needed.
5. **Brush** - A small- to medium-sized paintbrush will do fine. Whatever brush you get, make sure it is not too coarse.

While there are a few things you need in order to make your harvesting process a bit easier, the main thing to look out for is having a container, gloves, and a mask.

Harvesting Your Mushrooms

I know how excited you are at the moment, and you cannot wait to finally harvest your mushrooms. While it is practically as easy as pulling the mushroom from the substrate, you need to be sure you do it at the right time.

If you take a look at the terminology list, you will notice the word veil. As described there, it connects the cap to the stem, encasing and protecting the gills, which contain all the spores. So, when you monitor your growing mushrooms, you will have to keep a lookout for this veil. It is usually milky white, depending on the species of the mushroom.

The reason for this is pretty simple; you do not want the veil to break. If the veil breaks, the spores will soon be released. Timing differs between species, but once pinning has formed, your mushrooms will start to grow within a few days, leaving a very small window for harvesting before they mature completely and the veil breaks. The only thing that will make this monitoring process easier is experience.

When it is your first harvest, you might start the process too early due to being afraid the veils will break. Similarly, you might wake up the next morning and notice the veils broke already, leaving an oily and inky mess on your substrate, fruiting chamber, and other mushrooms. Do not worry if it doesn't work out perfectly the first time; you can still use them either way.

Harvesting will work pretty much the same no matter what type of fruiting chamber you used, even if you cultivated them outside. The same goes for the substrate; while a cake looks different from a tub full of substrate, the process works the same. So, let's get started with the process.

First, wait for the right time to harvest. Start getting all the harvesting equipment ready when you see the veils forming. Signs to look out for would be the cap of the mushroom changing from round to a more convex shape. The color of the mushroom will most likely start to change as well. Depending on the species, it will either become lighter or darker the more the cap protrudes from the stem. You will almost start to feel the tension on the veil as the cap turns more convex.

Sterilize all the containers and tools you will be using, just in case. Contamination of your mushrooms is practically impossible at this point, but who wants to work with dirty tools? Besides, if you want to keep growing after the harvest, you need to keep your area clean.

Once all the mushrooms are relatively the same size, and you feel like the veils could tear at any moment, you may begin the harvesting process. Some cultivators monitor each mushroom individually, harvesting them as they mature, leaving the others to grow further. Unfortunately, not everyone has the experience or time to do that. So, you can just wait till all of them seem ready for you. Start with a bigger mushroom, one that is easy to access without disturbing the others.

Here are the steps to follow:

1. Make sure all your equipment is sterilized and put on some fresh gloves.

2. Place your index finger and thumb at the base of the mushroom you chose for the easiest access. If there were none, just pick one at random.

3. You can start to gently pull and twist on the bottom of the stem. You will notice there are a few root-like protrusions from the base. That is what connects it to the mycelium network in your substrate. Try not to damage the network when pulling the mushrooms out.

4. If you have difficulty getting the mushroom to break away from the network, use your scissors to snip the roots.

5. The tweezers are there for the smaller or hard-to-reach mushrooms. Use them as an extension of your fingers to pull them from the network.

6. You will notice some material stuck at the bottom of the base of the mushroom you pulled out. It's usually leftover substrate, moss, or mycelium. Use the brush to remove it gently.

7. Place the mushroom in your sterile container and move on to the next one.

It is quite simple, isn't it? Something to look out for when pulling out the mushrooms is to not damage the veil if it is still intact. This goes for the ones in the sterile container and the ones you still need to harvest. Some people snip the base off the mushroom completely before placing it in the sterile container. While you can do that too if you want, there is really no point to it. Some people just do not like the thought of eating that part.

Continue Growing

What many people do not know is that you can continue to grow mushrooms off of the cake or substrate that you just harvested from. Remember, there is still a whole network of mycelium inside. So, as long as there are still nutrients and water, new mushrooms will start to grow again.

This is why it is important to keep everything as sterile as possible when harvesting. Now, you can take your water bottle, mist the container as you did before, and wait for the next harvest!

The network will keep growing new mushrooms every time you harvest them, given that there are enough nutrients left. Keep in mind that the risk for contamination of your network increases every time you harvest. The yield will become smaller and smaller as well if you keep on harvesting.

At that point, you can decide if it is worth the effort to keep the same network or just start a new one. At some point, however, it will die out due to a lack of nutrients. When that happens, you can remove the cake, sterilize the fruiting chamber, and start the whole process over again.

Do not throw the old network in the trash though; you can go and plant it somewhere outside so it can keep on growing.

Making Your Own Spore Kits

If you are looking to keep on growing new mushrooms, you will want to make your own spore kits. You can keep buying new spore syringes, especially if you want to try out a new species. However, why not just make your own if you are happy with the species you currently have?

You will need a few things, but let's start with the basic necessity of making a spore syringe.

Spore Prints

In order for you to be able to make your own spore syringes, you will have to make a print first. Well, there is the option of buying spore prints as well, but isn't the whole point of cultivating your own mushrooms to be self-sustaining?

Here is a list of what you will need:

1. Open cap mushroom - What this means is the veil will have to break naturally. What you can do is leave a couple of mushrooms in the FC while harvesting the others; wait for the veil to break and the cap to flatten out a bit. Pluck it and you will have yourself a mature mushroom.

2. A scalpel or sharp knife

3. A lighter

4. A still airbox (SAB) - You can use one of your unmodified monotubs—cut two holes on the one side, big enough for your hands and arms to get through. It will have to be a see-through one, big enough for you to be able to stick your arms in and work comfortably. The idea is to minimize airflow.

5. Rubbing alcohol

6. Sheets of clean paper or aluminum foil

7. A drinking glass - this will depend on the number of prints you want to make.

8. Tweezers

9. Small zip bag

Let's start with the process of making a spore print.

Sterilize the inside of your SAB with the rubbing alcohol, as well as everything you will be using. Place all the items inside the SAB except for the knife and lighter and close the lid.

Use the lighter to sterilize your scalpel/knife, same as with the needles when inoculating your grain. Let it cool off as you keep it in your hand. After that is done, insert your hands into the SAB and take the mushrooms you have saved for making spores. Cut off the stem of one right at the cap; try to do this without touching the gills/spores.

Place the cap gill side down on a piece of clean paper. Put a drinking glass over the cap to "seal" it. Do this for all the caps you have chosen. After about two hours, remove the glass and cap, throw the piece of paper away, and place it on a new piece of clean paper, with the glass over it again. The first spores are highly likely to be contaminated, which is why you throw that first print away. Now, you can leave them for around 12–24 hours. When the time comes, put on new gloves and remove the glasses and caps. You can cut out the prints left on the paper and fold them closed in the aluminum foil. Use the sterilized tweezers when doing this. Seal the prints in a zip bag and there you have it! A print that will last you quite a few years, given that you store it in a dark and cool place.

Spore Syringes

Now that you have your prints, you can make new syringes. Keep a print out for this while sealing and storing the others away. Here is a list of what you will need:

1. Empty syringes - this will depend on how many you want to make. Be sure they have needles attached.

2. Isopropyl alcohol

3. Sterile water

4. Your spore print

5. Lighter

6. Scalpel/knife

7. Tweezers

8. Shot glass

9. Still airbox (SAB)

Making the syringes is fairly easy. As with the prints, get everything sterilized with the alcohol and into the sterilized SAB. Use the lighter to sterilize the scalpel/knife and the needle of the first syringe. Insert your hands into the SAB and fill the shot glass with about 10 ml of sterile water.

Gently unwrap your spore print with the blade and tweezers. Pick the print up with the tweezers and start scraping some of the spores into the shot glass. The number of spores you scrape off will depend on the number of syringes you plan on making.

Take your syringe and place the needle in the water and give it a bit of a stir. Start filling up the syringe but not fully. Pull in some water and empty it back into the glass again a couple of times to make sure the spores are distributed evenly in the water. Fill the syringe, place the cap on the needle, and move on to the next syringe.

There, you have yourself a spore syringe! Easy right? If you used a fresh print that you made the same day, you can leave the syringe for about two hours at room temperature, so the spores can rehydrate. If it is an older print, you will have to leave it at room temperature to rehydrate for 24–72 hours, depending on how old it is. After that, you can place the syringes in your fridge; they will be viable for about six months. Some claim that it can be longer, but do not bank on that; you have the prints that will last years after all.

Storing Your Mushrooms

When it comes to storing your mushrooms, you will have to be careful, especially fresh ones. Everyone knows that fresh mushrooms are more potent, but due to the nature of fungi, they are really difficult to store fresh for longer periods of time. I would suggest storing your mushrooms in a variety of ways.

PSILOCYBIN MUSHROOMS

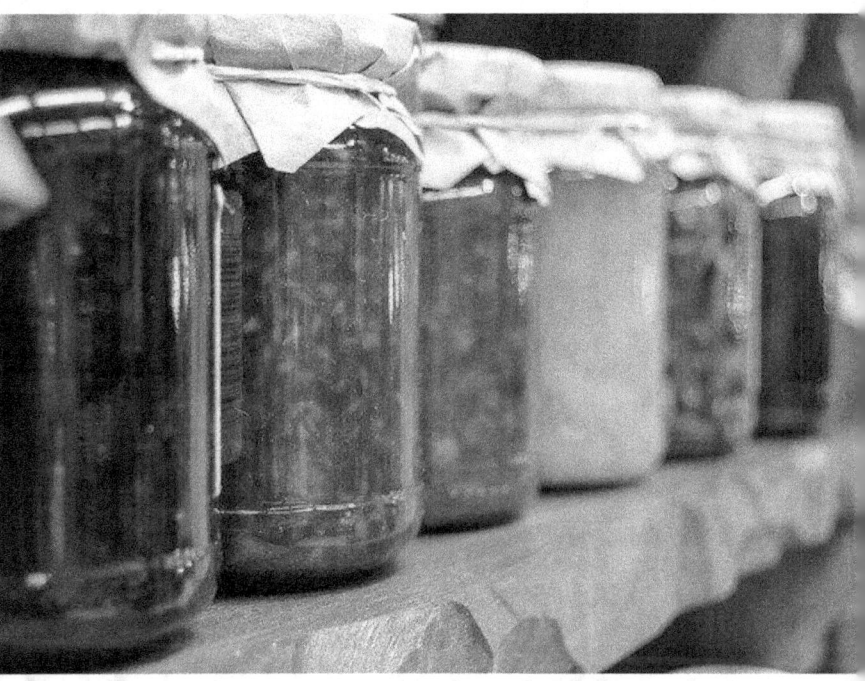

There are a few things you will have to do for each method of storage. Seeing as we just finished with all the harvesting, we can start with fresh storage methods first.

Fresh Storage

Contrary to what many people believe, sealing fresh mushrooms up in a container and placing them in a fridge will not keep them fresh for longer. In fact, they might even rot completely and turn into mush.

If you want to store fresh mushrooms that you just harvested, follow these few short steps. I would advise against trying to store bulk amounts of fresh psilocybin mushrooms.

- Rinse off the fresh mushrooms you want to store and dry them with a paper towel. Try to get as much of the surface moisture off the mushroom as possible without damaging it.

- Leave them out on a paper towel to dry for about 30 minutes.

- Take a brown paper bag and line it with pieces of paper towel.

- Place the mushrooms inside the bag but do not entirely seal it up.

- You can now place the bag in your fridge.

Fresh mushrooms do not last long, but in a paper bag, they will keep fresh for longer. The pieces of paper towel will keep most of the moisture away for a while. This method will ensure they stay fresh for about seven days. Keeping them in the fridge for longer than that will cause them to rot, very similar to the storage of any other mushroom.

Another option is freezing them; however, it will not go the way you think. Freezing a mushroom will cause the cells to rupture. When you thaw them out, you will be left with a black mush, which you cannot consume.

So, I would suggest freezing them and then consuming them while they are still frozen. Still, it is a very poor way to store them, so I will not suggest this as your main method of storage.

Drying

The best way to store your psilocybin mushrooms will be to dry them out first. This can be done in a few ways.

Food Dehydrator

The easiest way to dry and store them will be through using a food dehydrator. This is by far the most efficient way but not always the cheapest. There is quite a big variety of food dehydrators available on the market. It will all depend on the amount of money you are willing to spend.

One thing to keep in mind when drying your mushrooms, however, is that heat will destroy the psilocybin. So, if you do decide on getting a food dehydrator, you will have to get one that has the option to disable the heating element. If you cannot find one, you will have to modify it yourself, which can be dangerous.

You can simply place your mushrooms inside the food dehydrator and run it at the lowest setting. Run it as long as it takes, if there is no heat; the potency of your mushrooms will not be affected.

When you take out the mushrooms, they should be completely dried out. You should not be able to bend the stems or anything; they should break apart.

After that is done, you can store your mushrooms in a sealable container. You can throw in a few food-grade silica gel packs to keep any moisture from building up. You can vacuum pack your dried mushrooms as well. Keep the storage containers in a dry and dark place.

Drying Rack

You can build your own drying rack if you do not have a food dehydrator. Here is what you will need.

- A large grid, sheet pan, plate, or wire rack
- Kitchen towel or paper towels
- A fan

You can take your wire rack (or whichever flat surface object) and layer it with a towel/paper towel. Place it somewhere out of the way. Put the mushrooms on the towels and space them evenly apart so they do not stack over each other. Put the fan on its lowest setting to ensure you do not blow away your mushrooms.

That is it! You have your own drying rack. Depending on the humidity in the area where you live, it will take 1–5 days for them to dry out completely. Once again, be sure they are so dry that they fall apart in your hands when you try to break them.

Other Methods of Storage

There are a few other ways to store your mushrooms; however, they can sometimes get a bit complicated. Let's start with a method I prefer.

Capsules

Storing your mushrooms in capsule form can be a lengthy process, but it is worth it. You will have to dry them out first. Use a coffee grinder to grind the dried mushrooms into a very fine powder, as fine as possible. You can buy capsules from any store that sells medical and lab equipment. You will need a capsule filling machine as well.

Simply fill up the capsules with the fine powder, place the capsules in a sealable container with a food-grade silica gel pack, and you are done! The best part is you can swallow the capsules without tasting the mushrooms!

Honey

Through the ages, humans have used honey as a long-term storage medium. The same method can be used for your magic mushrooms. Here is how you can do it:

- You can slice up fresh mushrooms or dry them out and crush them.

- Throw some of the mushrooms into a sealable jar.

- Pour some honey over them and mix it all together.

- You can then start throwing in more mushrooms and more honey, mixing them every time. Be sure the mushrooms are evenly mixed in with the honey.

- Seal up the jar and store it in a cool and dark place.

This method works when storing your mushrooms for a few months; just check on the honey every now and then for mold. Dried mushrooms work better compared to fresh ones.

That's It!

There are quite a few ways to store your mushrooms after harvesting them; just make sure you do not try to store too much. In the end, you can only keep so much of it for so long before it all goes bad.

It is better to store a bit and then just grow fresh mushrooms again later on.

CHAPTER 5

USING PSILOCYBIN MUSHROOMS SAFELY

After going through all the effort of doing the research, building your setup, growing your mushrooms, and harvesting them… you probably want to eat them!

Before you do that, however, familiarize yourself with a few things. You do not want to jump down a rabbit hole without some form of assurance that you will end up safe on the other side.

There are a few things you will want to understand before munching down on those freshly harvested psilocybin mushrooms, so let's outline them quickly.

- How

- can go wrong

That is a basic outline you can follow before taking mushrooms. Let's go over some of them; it will go quick, I promise. Then you can get to have the satisfaction of enjoying your own hard work, safely.

Magic Mushroom Dosage Guide

The first thing to think about when consuming magic mushrooms is how much you actually want to consume. What type of experience are you looking for? If you are looking for a reasonably relaxed trip with moderate visuals, you don't want to pound 5 grams of mushrooms straight down your throat.

In order to understand what type of trip you will experience from certain dosages, I will lay out a guide for you. Keep in mind, these dosages are based on dried mushrooms. Fresh mushrooms are known to have a stronger potency to them, so beware.

Relaxed - If you want a pleasant, relaxed, and focused feeling with no visuals, you will want to consume 0.25 grams or less.

- **Light** - Having a generally relaxed feeling with some effects felt throughout your body will need more than 0.25 grams but no more than 1 gram.

- **Moderate** - If you are looking for a good trip with light visuals, you can try more than 1 gram. Do not consume more than 2.5 grams, however. This is the recommended dosage for beginners.

- **Strong** - Some of us are in it for a good visual trip, but we do not want to dive into existential dread just yet. For a great trip with good visuals, you will want to consume between 2.5 grams and 4 grams. Anything from this point on is not recommended for beginners.

- **Heavy** - This is where things start to get a little intense. The known threshold for a crazy trip is around 5 grams of psilocybin mushrooms. Do this only if you are prepared and have previous experience.

- **Cosmic** - Okay, let's face it… everyone wants to break through reality and enter a complete state of balance with matter and energy at some point in their psychedelic experiences. Dosages of 6 grams and up will usually achieve that, but 10 grams is the point of no return. If you consume 10 grams or more, you are in for one hell of a ride. You will have to be prepared spiritually, emotionally, psychologically, and physically. You will not be the same after coming back.

Something else to consider is the time it takes from consumption to hitting you, as well as the duration of the whole trip. This will largely depend on the actual dosage taken.

PSILOCYBIN MUSHROOMS

The usual time before onset is 20–40 minutes. This will depend on whether or not you ate anything before consuming the mushrooms. The duration of the trip itself can be from two hours to six hours. It might stretch to eight hours but that is usually only the aftereffects.

A big debate for beginners is when to take mushrooms and where to take mushrooms. Most people suggest taking them in the comfort of your own home, with no more than two or three friends present. You have to trust these friends as well, so they cannot be a bunch of random people. It makes the whole experience easier to handle.

You can consume them by yourself as well, but some people do not recommend that. At least have someone nearby if something happens. Before consuming mushrooms, have a specific intent in mind. Your state of mind and the intent with which you consume the mushrooms will have a big influence on the overall trip you experience. If you are having any negative thoughts or a general unstable state of mind, do not consume them without someone else present. That is how a bad trip becomes a six-hour hell.

You will also need to be aware that some people suffer from minor stomach cramps for about 30 minutes after consumption. This can really put a damper on your mood, but do not let it get to you. I am speaking from personal experience here. I once consumed around 3 grams of mushrooms and suffered severe cramps for about 2o minutes. I decided to lie down and try to ignore the cramps. A few minutes later the cramps faded away, and I had one of the best trips of my life!

You might also have a slight upset stomach the next day; this is different from person to person, however. Some people might not have any problems, while others will have a bad time in the toilet. Luckily it does not last long and usually only occurs with higher doses.

When a bad trip does occur, and it can happen, you will have to try and remain calm. It can be quite difficult, especially when taking more than 5 grams. Try to remember that you are under the influence of something you consumed. Remember that there is a time limit to how long it will last and that it will not be forever. Doing that will calm you down and can turn a personal nightmare into a profound experience.

Music can change your trip for better or worse. There is a reason people enjoy going to concerts while tripping on mushrooms. If you choose a good playlist, your trip can be magical. Try to make a playlist of music before actually consuming the mushrooms.

Different Consumption Methods

Some people enjoy eating their mushrooms as is. It really is not for everyone, and there is nothing wrong with that! There are multiple ways you can consume magic mushrooms, so let's take a look at some of them.

Raw - As I said, some people do not mind the taste. I myself am not a fan of the taste at all, but it isn't that bad. What you can do is crush up the mushrooms, throw them into your mouth, and gulp down with some water.

Mix - Some people will take the mushrooms and mix them with something edible. Keep in mind that heat destroys psilocybin, so baking them with cookies is not a good idea. What you can do, however, is mix it in with some yogurt, fruit, or cereal. I like making a peanut butter sandwich and sprinkle some on there, works like a charm.

Tea - You will find that many mushroom enthusiasts actually make tea with their mushrooms. All you need for a basic tea is some hot water, ginger, mushrooms, and honey. Grind up the mushrooms and pour them into a cup and add ginger and honey. Pour some hot water (not boiling hot) into the cup and stir. You can customize the tea as you like; just make sure that the water is not too hot when making it. The onset of the effects is usually much quicker when drinking mushrooms in tea form.

Capsules - Using capsules can be quite interesting. You will not have the bad taste, and you have the added benefit of the exact dosage. Due to the fact that you can get capsules of varying sizes, you can load up capsules for a microdose of 0.10–0.25 grams. Or you can load up bigger capsules with 1 gram. You will be able to drink as many as you want the dosage to be with water.

There you have the basics of how to consume your mushrooms and how to do so safely! So, go and enjoy your hard labor!

CHAPTER 6: GENERAL TIPS

In this chapter, I will be pointing out a few mistakes that beginners might make with their first cultivation. We will also be going over what might go wrong when cultivating your mushrooms, such as pests and diseases that might influence your mushrooms.

Pest, Contamination, and Disease Control

No matter what we do, sometimes we have to deal with either contamination or pests.

Pests

There are in general only four pests to worry about when cultivating mushrooms:

- Cecid fly
- Sciarid fly
- Phorid fly
- Fungus mites

When you sterilize your whole environment as well as your substrates, you will have very little to no chance of seeing any of these pests interfere with your cultivation. This is especially true when dealing with an indoor FC, but they are much more likely to appear in outdoor cultivation areas. So, how do you prevent and treat them?

You will immediately start to notice when there are flies in your FC. When this happens, it can be pretty much guaranteed that they have already spawned their larvae in your substrate. There is not much you can do when this happens. The best method is to make sure everything is sterilized beforehand so that no pests come with your substrate in the first place. You can also have a casing layer of coffee or tobacco over your substrate; the flies will not come near it.

You do not want to spray any toxic chemicals either, so the best way to counter the flies is by introducing natural predators. Venus flytraps and praying mantises will be your only defense in this case.

PSILOCYBIN MUSHROOMS

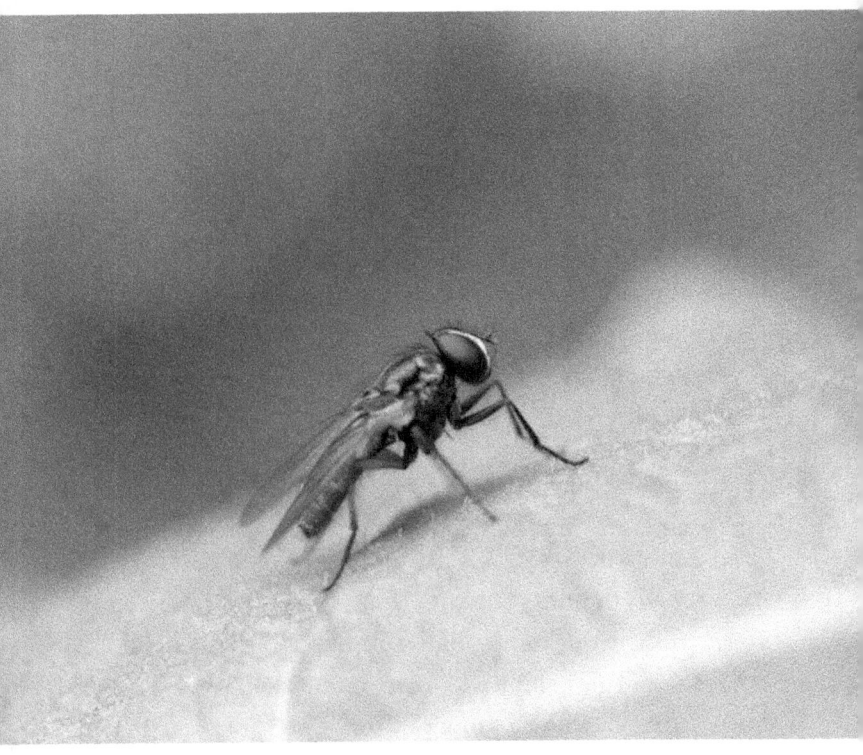

Fungus mites are very small white-yellow creatures that can infest your FC. These are generally prevented through proper sterilization. If you do spot them, however, you do not have to worry. Most of them are not harmful to your mushrooms, while some might feed on the mycelium network. You can simply mix a bit of alcohol, lemon juice, and water to spray your mushrooms with. It should take care of the problem. No one really wants little white bugs crawling over their mushrooms anyway.

Contamination and Disease

There are quite a few contaminants that might influence your mushroom cultivation. The only way to prevent these is through proper sterilization. You will have to throw everything away and start over if these are picked up during cultivation.

Here we will make a list of the most likely contaminants that can enter your cultivation journey.

- **Wet spot/sour rot** - This usually happens during the mycelium colonization phase of your grain. A dull gray slime will form in the pack/jar, which will reek with a sour odor. The grain will look excessively wet.

- **Bacterial blotch** - When yellowish-brown lesions form on your mushroom caps, bacterial blotch has contaminated the FC. This can happen if the substrate was not sterilized properly and the humidity is too high in the FC. Remember that fresh air is a key component in cultivating mushrooms.

- **Cobweb mold** - if you see a strange cotton/cobweb-like mycelium grow over your mushrooms and substrate, it is contaminated. The color is darker than psilocybin mushroom mycelium and spreads lightning-fast, like in a few hours. Make sure the FC gets enough fresh air.

- **Green mold** - This is a very aggressive mold and will cause your mushrooms to rot. The only prevention is proper sterilization of all surfaces and tools.

- **Pink mold** - If you see a pink mold form, throw everything away immediately. It usually starts with the poly-fill filters and spreads to your FC. So, make sure you replace the filters and spray them properly with disinfectant.

- **Blue mold** - If a sticky blue mold forms over your substrate, you will have to throw it out, unfortunately. Prevention is the same as with the others—a sanitary workspace and sterile equipment/substrate.

- **Black mold** - If you spot this, be sure to handle it gently. You will have to wear a mask as the spores are toxic when inhaled. Throw everything out and wipe down the entire room/workspace.

Some Tips

- Always clean everything. If you can't remember if you sterilized something, do it again just in case.

- Try to use presterilized grain packs that you can buy online or from shops in your area. It makes the beginner cultivator's life much easier.

- If you see any sticky mold and smell weird odors, you can assume everything is contaminated and start over.

- The internet is your friend; there are a lot of websites and forums dedicated to helping you cultivate mushrooms.

- If the veils of your mushrooms broke and the spores have been released, you can still harvest your mushrooms. Just wash them off.

- If you doubt what species to start with, go with *Psilocybe cubensis*. It is the most popular starter mushroom.

- If you do not see anything happen in your FC after a week, just give it a bit more time, and do not stop misting. The mycelium can sometimes take its time.

- Go with the simplest options first. You do not have to start out with a complicated setup.

- When eating your new mushrooms for the first time, test out the waters first. You can have just a little bit to see exactly how potent they turned out. While most species have a set potency level, they can still vary a lot.

- Enjoy cultivating your own psilocybe mushrooms! It is a fun experience, especially when doing it with a partner. So, enjoy every moment.

CONCLUSION

I hope that after reading this, you will be confident enough to approach your first cultivation experience with a smile and reassurance.

Growing psilocybin mushrooms is really not that difficult, as long as you pay attention and clean everything properly. Psilocybin mushrooms have been with humanity since the beginning. We started with foraging for them, and now we are cultivating them.

The experience of cultivating your own mushrooms and then enjoying the mind-blowing results is something everyone should try at least once.

So, why are you still here? Go and grow your own psychedelic experience!

PSILOCYBIN MUSHROOMS

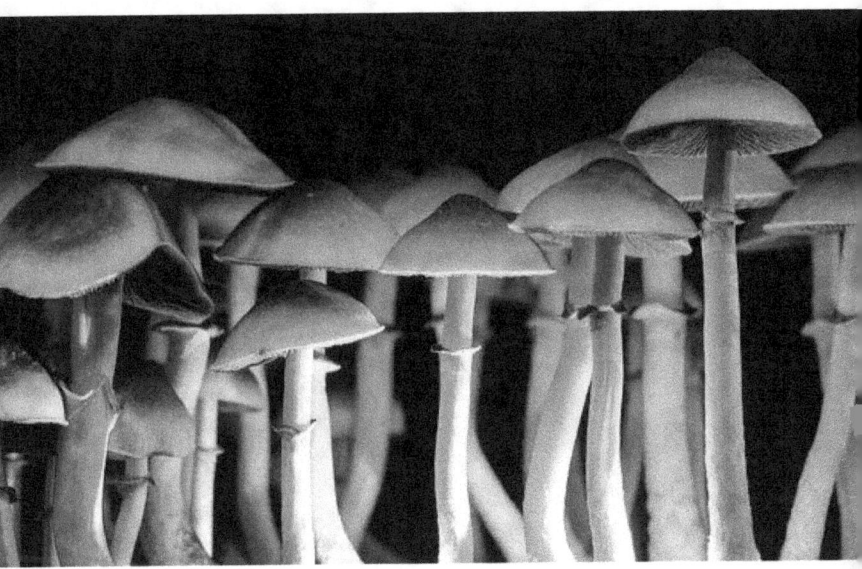

www.ingramcontent.com/pod-product-compliance
Lightning Source LLC
Chambersburg PA
CBHW050319120526
44592CB00014B/1977